MUSCLE TESTING

A Concise Manual

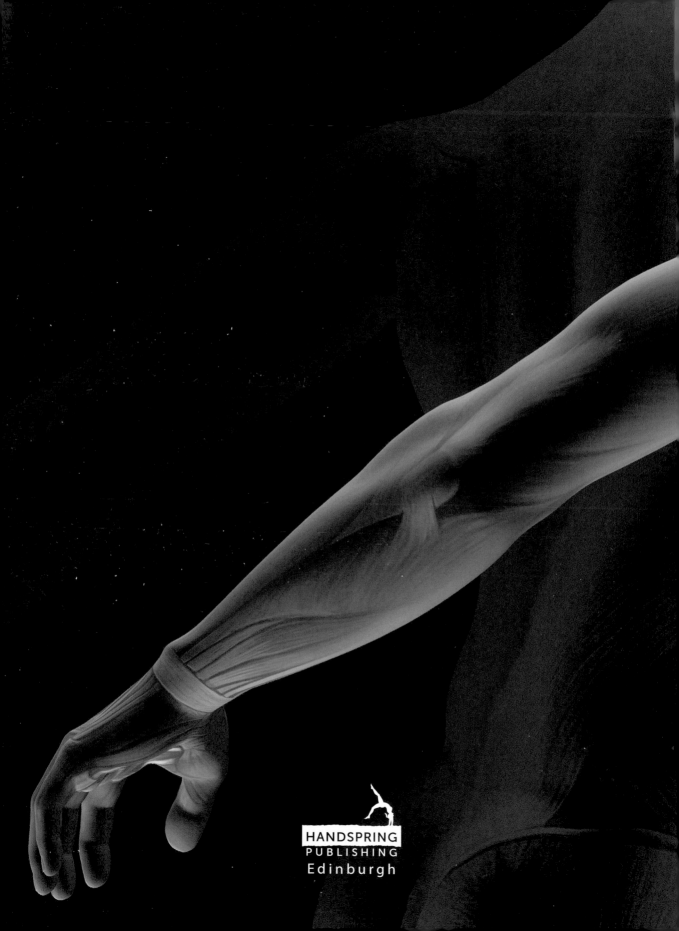

HANDSPRING
PUBLISHING
Edinburgh

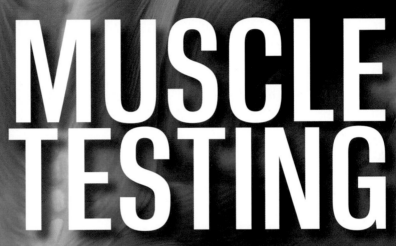

MUSCLE TESTING
A Concise Manual

Earle Abrahamson
Jane Langston

Forewords by
David H. Perrin
Ian McCarthy

HANDSPRING PUBLISHING LIMITED
The Old Manse, Fountainhall,
Pencaitland, East Lothian
EH34 5EY, Scotland
Tel: +44 1875 341 859
Website: www.handspringpublishing.com

First published 2019 in the United Kingdom by Handspring Publishing

ISBN 978-1-912085-65-1
ISBN (Kindle ebook) 978-1-912085-66-8
British Library Cataloguing in Publication Data
A catalogue record for this book is available from the British Library

Library of Congress Cataloguing in Publication Data
A catalog record for this book is available from the Library of Congress

Notice
Neither the Publisher nor the Authors assume any responsibility for any loss or injury and/or damage to persons or property arising out of or relating to any use of the material contained in this book. It is the responsibility of the treating practitioner, relying on independent expertise and knowledge of the patient, to determine the best treatment and method of application for the patient.

Commissioning Editor Mary Law
Project Manager Morven Dean
Copy Editor Stephanie Pickering
Designer Bruce Hogarth
Photographer Sue Magar
Indexer Aptara
Typesetter DSM Soft, India
Printer Replika, India

The
Publisher's
policy is to use
paper manufactured
from sustainable forests

CONTENTS

Section THREE
GAIT TESTING   262

How to access the online videos

Within this book you will find QR codes that will take you to instructional videos that accompany the text. These QR codes can be scanned with a smart phone using an app, and many free apps are available to download. If you are using an iPad or iPhone running the latest software (iOS 11 or higher) then no additional app is required. Simply open your camera and point it at the code (no need to take a picture). A notification should pop down from the top and then tap that and you will be taken to the video.

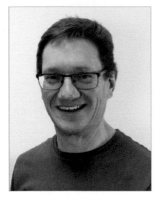

Earle Abrahamson BPhysEd, BAHons, MA, PFHEA
Chair, Massage Training Institute
Vice-Chair, General Council for Massage Therapies
Elected Professional Subject Board member, Complementary and
Natural Healthcare Council

Earle Abrahamson holds qualifications in sports and human movement sciences,
clinical psychology, and pedagogy. He is a Principal Fellow of Advanced HE, Inaugural
ISSoTL Fellow, and Programme Leader/Senior Lecturer in Sports Therapy at the University
of East London, UK. He has over 20 years of experience in education and clinical practice
and leads the functional anatomy modules on the Sports Therapy programme at the
University of East London. Earle is director at Learn Anatomy Ltd and Hands-On Training
Ltd. Earle is a practicing soft tissue therapist who actively uses muscle testing to assess
and treat a wide range of injuries and pathologies.

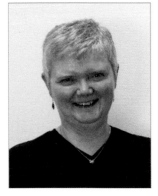

Jane Langston
Fellow of the Institute of Biomedical Science (Haematology)
Committee Member, General Council for Massage Therapies
Amatsu Ambassador, Amatsu Therapy International (UK)
Managing Director, Learn Anatomy Ltd and Amatsu Training
School Ltd (Bury St Edmunds).

Jane Langston worked for over 20 years in haematology and blood transfusion laboratories
within the UK National Health Service. She went on to spend another 20 years developing
her skills as an Amatsu practitioner in a busy clinic in Hertfordshire. Jane is a teacher of
Amatsu soft tissue therapy and anatomy and physiology and is a director of Amatsu
Training School Ltd and Learn Anatomy Ltd. Jane is an Amatsu therapy representative
on the General Council for Soft Tissue Therapies and is an Amatsu advisor to the British
Register for Complementary Therapies. As a result of many years of teaching she
understands that students need good strategies to help them learn, retain, and apply
anatomical studies.

Writing a text requires patience, support, and a vision to communicate information to a diverse audience. The process is arduous, often resulting in difficult periods of rethinking ideas, framing of words and concepts, and re-reading text from different perspectives. It is during these complex and difficult times that the closeness and supportive relationship of significant others becomes paramount.

My wife, Emma, who lovingly gave me space to think and create, and taught me resolve and perseverance, I thank you dearly. My wonderful sons, Benjamin and Oliver, who inquisitively watched me write and asked interesting questions about the content and purpose of the book, I thank you for your understanding, inspiration, and enabling me to encourage you to follow a similar path. My brother, Michael, who inspired me to think big and live the moment, I thank you for your continued words of wisdom.

To my co-author Jane, thank you for encouraging me to continue the writing process and using our collective skills to create a text for practice. I thank you for your vision, support, and ability to promote our work through social media and workshops.

To the ever-increasing community of practitioners, who taught me how to use my knowledge for learning, I greatly appreciate your input, advice, and sharing of useful tips. This book has taught me to phrase ideas in a succinct way and build an appreciation for capturing essential information. To the team at Handspring

Publishing, who caringly guided us through the process and exercised patience and commitment to the final product, I thank you sincerely.

Finally, I dedicate this book to my late parents, who taught me to pursue my dreams, and believe in myself.

Earle Abrahamson

The ability to properly assess a client in a scientific, yet holistic manner has always been my goal and has allowed me the privilege of working with some amazing and inspiring people. I must, therefore, give thanks to all my teachers, students, and clients who have pushed my curiosity to its outer limits and beyond in the clinic and training rooms of Amatsu Soft Tissue Therapy.

For teamwork, co-operation and partnership, I thank my co-author, Earle Abrahamson, without whom I could not have written this text. I would like to thank our model, Mark Langston. This completed book could not have been produced without the talent of our photographer, Sue Magar, and the creativity and belief of the whole Handspring Publishing team, so thank you all.

Finally, and most importantly, my family have always been hugely accommodating of my yearning to learn, so I thank my husband, Mark, and my son, David, for their love and unfailing support.

Jane Langston

As a student of athletic training in the 1970s, I acquired a book titled *Physical Examination of the Spine and Extremities* by Stanley Hoppenfeld. The book transformed the way I learned, practiced, and taught for decades. I believe *Muscle Testing – A Concise Manual* by Earle Abrahamson and Jane Langston will have the same transformative impact on today's students of the health professions.

A sound understanding of functional anatomy serves as the foundation for muscle testing – and indeed all that we undertake in the rehabilitation sciences. Section 1 of the book provides an overview of musculoskeletal anatomy, testing, and palpation, including a description of active, passive, and resistive forms of motion and the concave and convex rule of joint motion. The physiology of muscle contraction is then reviewed as an introduction to the concepts of isometric and isotonic manual muscle testing. Next, the role of palpation in the location of soft tissue structures is presented, with useful hints to facilitate development of palpation skills provided. Section 1 concludes with an overview of how students can most effectively use the book, and encourages the learner to consider three essential learning points: anatomy, function, and individual versus group muscle testing. An important checklist of questions to be contemplated by the examiner for each muscle test is provided.

Section 2 presents muscle tests by region for 60 muscles of the head and neck, shoulder and elbow, forearm and wrist, torso and trunk, pelvis, thigh and knee, and lower leg, ankle, and foot. For each muscle, an anatomical overview and orientation of the muscle with its associated action, arterial and nerve supply are presented. Especially useful clinical facts, focusing on clinical assessments and structural alignments, are provided for each muscle. Guidelines for locating and palpating each muscle are provided, with special emphasis on understanding both the surface and deeper anatomical orientations. The manual muscle test itself is then presented, including considerations for patient positioning, and force generation and stabilization techniques, with graded, manual, and kinesiological perspectives provided.

The functional application of muscle testing is further brought to life in Section 3, which introduces gait testing for contralateral shoulder and hip flexor, extensor, abductor, adductor, contralateral psoas and pectoralis major, and contralateral gluteus and abdominal muscle groups. The authors astutely underscore the complexity of gait and locomotion activities that require a combination of facilitation, inhibition, isometric and eccentric muscle contraction. The contralateral gait tests, which use the major muscles in the upper and lower body that initiate walking movement, are illustrated with appropriate position, test, and stabilization techniques.

Muscle Testing – A Concise Manual is supported by high quality anatomical illustrations and photography. To supplement these illustrations, the techniques presented throughout the text are accompanied by video recordings accessible by code at the conclusion of each section. The book is organized in a manner supported by sound pedagogical principles that facilitate classroom and laboratory instruction. It will serve as an essential textbook for students and an ongoing reference for practicing clinicians for years to come. I am delighted to witness its introduction into the muscle testing literature, and pleased to provide this Foreword in support of its release to the community of health professions faculty, students, and clinicians.

David H. Perrin PhD, FACSM,
FNATA, FNAK
Dean and Professor
College of Health
University of Utah
Salt Lake City, Utah, USA

After graduating from my undergraduate degree, I had the good fortune to spend two amazing years at Stanford University Sports Medicine, in California. Within that multidisciplinary environment, I was gifted many clinical pearls from my mentors. There was, however, one piece of advice that unquestionably had the most profound impact on my career and I would like to share that same advice with you.

With an ever-increasing abundance of continuing professional development courses, textbooks, and online programs, it is difficult to know how best to utilize our time and energy in order to become truly great clinicians. Furthermore, from a business perspective, we all need a skill set, a service, or a knowledge base that sets us apart from our peers. This is a key aspect to any established business after all. Nonetheless, in order to be successful in our fields as health practitioners, we must strive to master three critically important clinical skills.

Firstly, we must be effective communicators in the presence of our patients to both extract important subjective information and also educate them on their treatment journey. Secondly, we should be able accurately to assess and diagnose our patients' dysfunctions and subsequent pains. Lastly, a skilled practitioner should possess a diverse treatment "tool box" to provide targeted and clinically appropriate treatments to a multitude of patient scenarios. But only one of these skills is paramount, and that is our assessment skills.

Put simply, you can be a highly efficient communicator but communicate the wrong information. Similarly, you may possess an impressive array of treatment techniques and modalities but treat the wrong area. The assessment is without any doubt the most crucial part of our profession and should be treated as such by investing more of our time and energy in it. I am referring to this in terms of self-directed learning and continuing professional development. I know Earle and Jane share this viewpoint and they have, therefore, carefully created Muscle Testing – a concise manual to help us connect our anatomical knowledge with the applied practice of manual muscle testing.

Nine years into my career in private practice, my conviction of the importance of our assessment skills has only further solidified. All too frequently I meet desperate patients at my clinic who have bounced from therapist to therapist, only finding short-term relief of symptoms. Being able to precisely identify a patient's underlying root dysfunction will have the greatest impact on the patient's clinical outcomes. The foundation of identifying any local or global somatic dysfunctions can be traced back to manual muscle testing. Educating ourselves with the information in *Muscle Testing – A Concise Manual* is a key foundation in honing the necessary assessment skills to be truly great practitioners. This book is a clear, concise, and well illustrated resource for both established professionals and health care students.

Ian McCarthy MSc Ost, GSR, CSCS
Vancouver Osteopathy Centre
Vancouver, BC, Canada

The musculoskeletal system is often taken for granted when it appears to work effortlessly. Human movement is a complex collection of interactions of body tissues and its collective function relies on the fine motor control of countless structures. It is only when function becomes dysfunction that the true complexity of the human movement machine is experienced.

Muscle testing is often part of a suite of therapeutic skills taught and practiced in multiple ways. Previously published texts on the subject provide analysis of muscle function and often illustrate only a single approach to testing. As educators it is important for us to understand how practitioners and students use information and what information becomes meaningful in their practices and learning. Drawing inspiration from the *Muscle Manual* by Nikita A. Vizniak, this book will serve as a companion to therapists, providing easily digestible text which highlights key points and presents multiple approaches to muscle testing.

We have analyzed how best to make information accessible to different audiences, and have organized our book accordingly. Each chapter contains drawings, photographs, and links to video material to accommodate all learning styles. Our approach will remind the reader about muscle anatomy, palpatory techniques, and clinical facts.

One of our aims has been to consider muscle testing in the context of our understanding of the role of fascia and biotensegrity. Thus each muscle has its actions listed, including those that occur when it is eccentrically contracted – a consideration omitted from the majority of textbooks and much needed when thinking about musculoskeletal function and dysfunction. Our understanding and experience of different approaches to soft tissue therapy and musculoskeletal management have inspired the creation of this text, to help improve practices and indeed to transform them.

We use text and illustrations to demonstrate correct positioning of the patient, which is crucial to achieving effective and accurate muscle testing within a practice-based environment. Muscle testing is often considered as a pre-treatment assessment technique, yet these tests can and should be used throughout a treatment to assess muscle activation and treatment impact. The sequencing of chapters into functional areas of the body emphasizes the importance of integrating muscle tests to assess function and dysfunction. The concluding chapters connect the complexity of human movement by considering dynamic patterns of locomotor control in the form of gait testing. An alphabetical index allows for quick location of details of specific muscles. A glossary provides definitions of words and phrases that may be unfamiliar to the reader.

We have aimed to create a text that captures the anatomy of muscle testing in a way that can be used to reinforce the understanding of the relationship between structure and function. We are grateful to the many colleagues who read the original book proposal and the subsequent manuscript and who provided insightful comments to help us develop the content. We hope our book will be used by both students and practitioners and will remain a faithful friend throughout their working life.

Finally we feel honored that David H. Perrin and Ian McCarthy agreed to contribute forewords. Both are leading educators and practitioners who can articulate the importance of using muscle testing in practical and academic environments.

Earle Abrahamson
Jane Langston
June 2019

References

Vizniak NA (2012) *Muscle manual*, Canada: Professional Health Systems Inc.

abduct move a limb away from the midline of the body

adduct move a limb toward the midline of the body

AIIS anterior inferior iliac spine

anterior front of body

ASIS anterior superior iliac spine

biotensegrity a structural design principle that describes a relationship between every part of an organism and the mechanical system that integrates them into a complete functional unit

concentric a type of isotonic muscle contraction wherein the muscle shortens under tension

connective tissue tissue that connects, supports, binds, or separates other tissues or organs

contralateral opposite side of the body

costal pertaining to the ribs

distal away from the point of attachment

dorsiflex movement of toes and/or ankle upward toward the shin

dynamic a force causing movement at a joint

dysfunction abnormality or impairment of function

eccentric a type of isotonic muscle contraction wherein the muscle lengthens under tension

elasticity (muscle) the ability of a muscle to return to its original length after being stretched

electromyography (EMG) a diagnostic procedure to assess the health of muscles and the nerve cells that control them (motor neurons)

excitability (muscle) the ability of a muscle to respond to a nerve or hormonal impulse which enables muscle regulation

extension straightening a limb or increasing the angle of a joint

fascia an interwoven system of connective tissue found throughout the body. Fascia helps to support and protect muscles and organs and connects body regions

flexion the bending of a limb or decreasing the angle of a joint

gait cycle starts when one foot makes contact with the ground and ends when that same foot contacts the ground again. The cycle can be broken down into various phases and periods to determine normative and abnormal gait

GHJ (glenohumeral joint) shoulder joint

hypertonic state of abnormally high muscle tone

hypotonic state of low muscle tone

inferior toward the feet

infra- pertaining to inferior

insertion the attachment of a muscle to a bone. The insertion moves with the muscle contraction

ipsilateral pertaining to the same side of the body

isometric tension is developed within the muscle without contraction of the muscle

isotonic contractions generate force by changing the length of the muscle

ITB (iliotibial band) tight fibrous connective tissue joining the hip to the knee found on the lateral (outside) aspect of the thigh

kinematics the study of motion of objects

kinesiology the study of the mechanics of body movement

lateral an anatomical reference term meaning toward the outside of the body

morphology the study of body shape

neurovascular pertaining to the nerve and blood supply of a tissue

origin the attachment of a muscle to a bone. The attachment is usually fixed during muscle contraction

palpation the process of using one's hands to check the body, especially while perceiving/diagnosing a disease or illness

patellofemoral syndrome a painful condition that affects the inner aspect of the knee where the patella is compressed against the femur. This condition is aggravated by physical activity or prolonged sitting

PIIS posterior inferior iliac spine

piriformis syndrome a condition that arises when the sciatic nerve branches are compressed by the piriformis muscle. This can lead to radiating pain or loss of feeling down the back of the thigh and leg

plantarflex movement at the ankle such that the toes move toward the floor or point toes downward

posterior pertaining to the back of the body

postural fatigue syndrome a condition that arises from incorrect use of the body posture and leads to tiredness or stiffness in postural muscles

prone lying face down

proximal a point situated closer to the attachment of structure or body segment

PSIS posterior superior iliac spine

quadrilateral space syndrome or quadrangular space syndrome a rotator cuff denervation syndrome in which the axillary nerve is compressed at the quadrilateral space of the rotator cuff

ROM (range of motion) can be divided into active range, passive range, resisted range

SCM sternocleidomastoid muscle

SIJ sacroiliac joint

"SITS" muscles an acronym for the group of rotator cuff muscles (Supraspinatus, Infraspinatus, Teres minor and Subscapularis)

static usually pertains to a stretch wherein there is limited movement of the body

superior toward the head

supine lying face up

supra- relating to superior

TFL tensor fasciae latae muscle

thenar relating to the intrinsic group of muscles located on the thumb side of the palm of the hand

thoracic outlet syndrome a group of disorders that occur when blood vessels or nerves in the space between the clavicle and first rib (thoracic outlet) are compressed. This can cause pain in the shoulders and neck and numbness in the fingers

volar relating to the palm of the hand or sole of the foot

VMO (vastus medialis obliquus) the portion of muscle superior to the knee on the medial aspect is sometimes referred to as the VMO

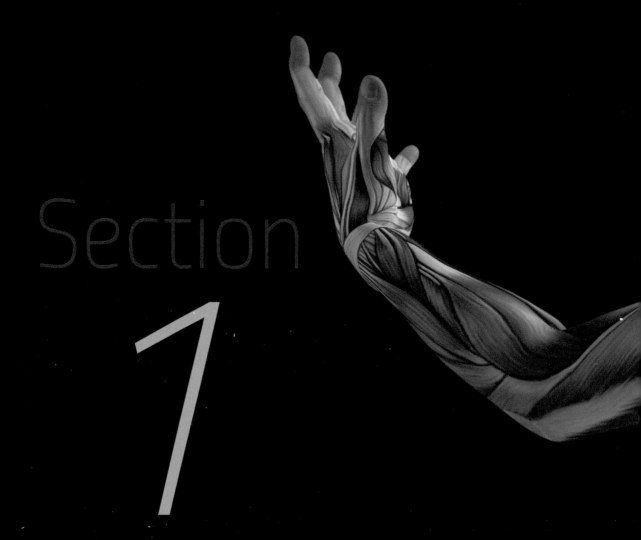

Section

1

INTRODUCTION

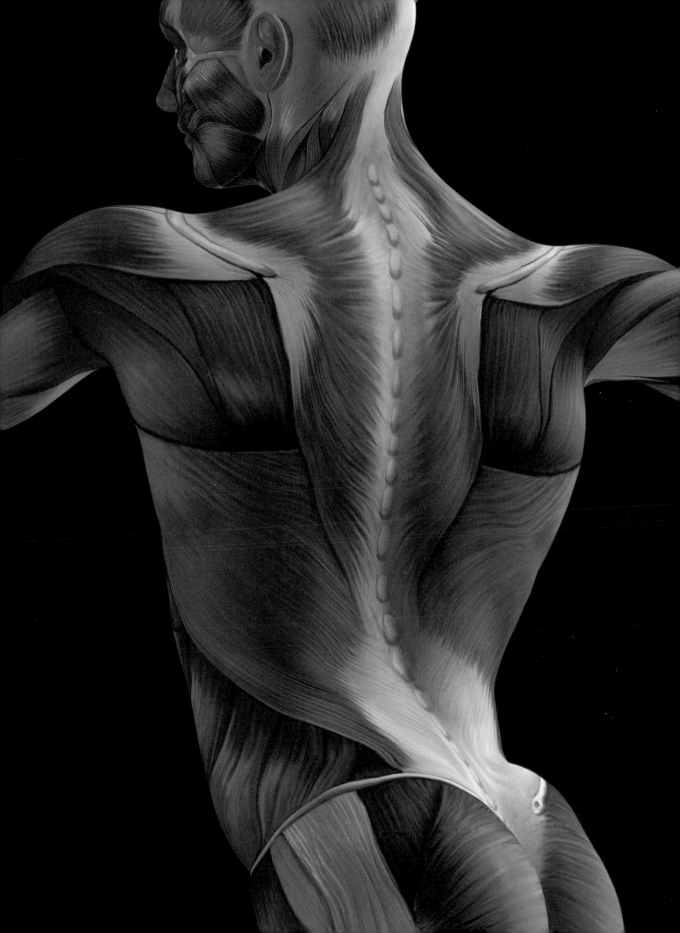

Introduction and principles of muscle testing

From sarcomere to muscle belly, the study of human muscles is a fascinating journey in and through structure and function. With over 800 muscles, the human body moves in complex ways, performs intricate tasks, and adapts to changes in the environment. The muscular system provides an important structural component for human function and enables us to maintain a bipedal posture. This unique ability to stand on two limbs separates humans from the other species. Through evolution we have learned to adapt, develop, grow, and move in ways that support the function and workings of the body. These movement patterns, accompanied by the interrelationship of body systems, not only depict function but equally monitor dysfunction. How do we know when our function is impaired? What specific metrics can we use to assess, treat, and rehabilitate musculoskeletal dysfunction? How does anatomical appreciation of muscle structure heighten understanding of dysfunction and pathology?

The inspiration for this book is drawn from the muscle manual by Vizniak (2012), who created a text that serves to inform, illustrate, and educate practitioners about muscle structure and function. Extending the philosophy of the Vizniak text, this concise manual aims to not only connect anatomy with muscle testing, but more importantly, provide a reference for understanding how structure relates to function, and how by knowing function we can learn structural configurations. Often muscular anatomy is taught as a dry study whereby each muscle is painstakingly studied, with the learner being expected to cite origin, insertion, action, nerve supply, and blood supply. This commonly used approach may not necessarily aid understanding of muscle function, nor does it relate to muscular positioning. Through muscle testing, one is better equipped to consider how muscles work individually and in working groups. It is the knowledge of symmetrical movement, range of motion, contractile patterns, resistance, and gravity that provides the fuller picture for muscle function and dysfunction.

Overview of musculoskeletal anatomy, testing, and palpation

Range of motion

Muscles control how joints move across planes and axes and as such have a specific movement range. Movement is complicated with many muscles producing action across different planes and axes, some helping each other to fine-tune the direction and amplitude of the movement.

Movement can best be understood as:

- Active, where the client performs the movement unaided
- Passive, where the examiner moves the limb into a final position
- Resisted, where the examiner applies resistance whilst the client moves the limb.

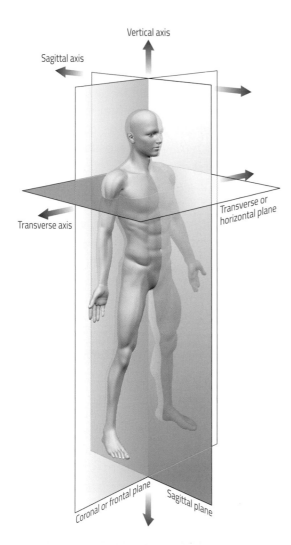

Vertical axis

Sagittal axis

Transverse or horizontal plane

Transverse axis

Coronal or frontal plane

Sagittal plane

Planes and axes of motion

The movement of joints provides a landscape for considering the shape of bones and restrictions in movement ranges. To better explain the way in which joints move, it is useful to consider the concave and convex rule.

Concave and convex rule of joint movement

Simply put, each joint has a concave as well as a convex surface. Take, for example, the elbow joint complex. If we focus on the hinge joint mechanics, we can see that part of the joint comprises the trochlear notch on the ulna, articulating with the trochlea of the humerus. The trochlear notch is concave, whilst the trochlea is convex. The important learning point to consider is which part of the bone moves to produce the action. Here the trochlear notch moves over the trochlea. As the trochlear notch moves upward, so does the forearm, enabling flexion of the joint. In other words, if the concave part moves, it moves in the same direction as the limb.

Way to remember this: "People in a cave stay together."

In the shoulder joint we have a convex humeral head, moving across a shallow concave glenoid fossa. As the head of the humerus moves downwards in the socket, the arm moves up. Relating this to the concave and convex rule – if the convex surface moves it moves in the opposite direction to the one in which the limb moves.

Irrespective of the method used, each movement presents relevant information regarding the function of joints and soft tissues. This enables the examiner to make informed decisions about structural inadequacies.

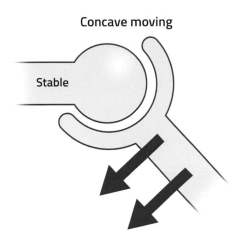

Concave moving

Stable

Concave movement at the elbow joint complex

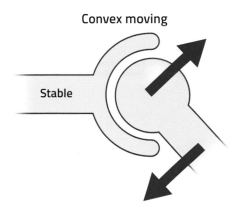

Convex moving

Stable

Convex movement at the glenohumeral joint

This is important for functional joint kinematics or the ability of the joint to work efficiently.

When assessing joint ROM, remember to consider the full range and identify any restrictive components. This will assist in a functional analysis of the joint and provide a road map for further assessment, treatment and rehabilitation.

Table 1 will help you revisit the range of motion for different joints. Use the table to consider the normal ranges, and potential restrictions with a range for all movements (i.e. active, passive, and resisted).

Assessing and testing muscle activation and strength

For a muscle to work, it needs to become excited. This may sound strange, but excitability is the unique ability of skeletal muscle to respond to a nerve impulse. Muscles are complex structures that contract and lengthen to produce movement. Anatomically speaking,

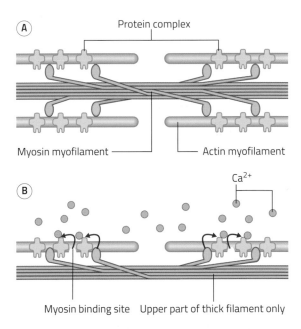

Ⓐ Protein complex

Myosin myofilament — Actin myofilament

Ⓑ Ca^{2+}

Myosin binding site   Upper part of thick filament only

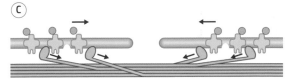

Ⓒ

Sliding filament theory

Table 1   Range of motion

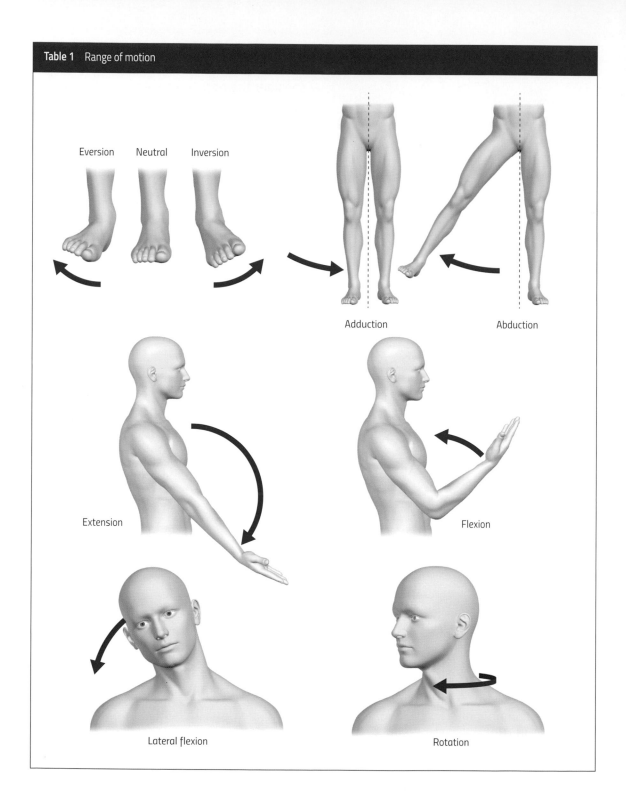

Eversion   Neutral   Inversion

Adduction

Abduction

Extension

Flexion

Lateral flexion

Rotation

Table 1 continued

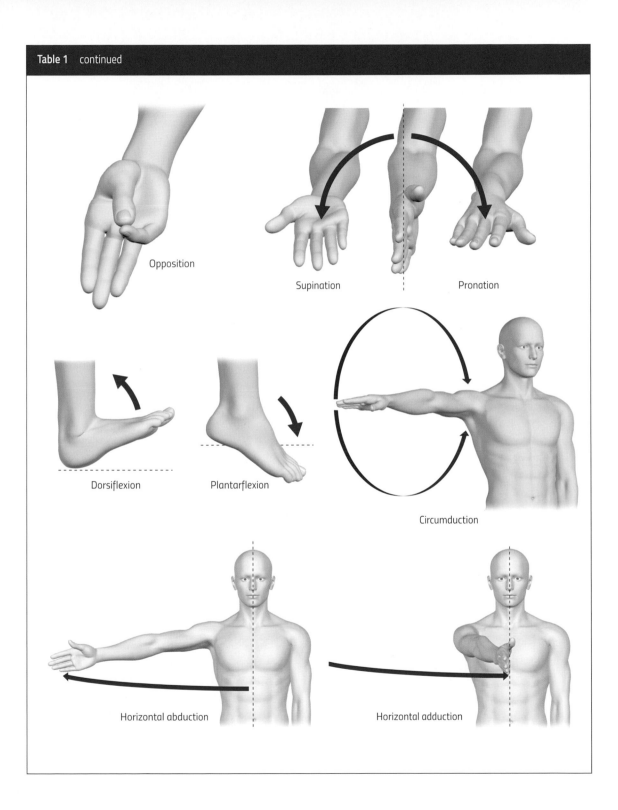

Opposition

Supination

Pronation

Dorsiflexion

Plantarflexion

Circumduction

Horizontal abduction

Horizontal adduction

Table 1 continued		
Motion	**Plane**	**Axis**
Flexion/extension	Sagittal	Horizontal/frontal
Abduction/adduction Lateral flexion Inversion/eversion	Frontal	Anterior/posterior
Internal and external rotation Horizontal flexion Supination/pronation	Transverse	Vertical/longitudinal

the gross functional contractile unit consists of the muscle and the associated soft tissues including connective tissue, tendons, and nerve supply. The sliding filament theory explains the physiological responses and relates the binding and unbinding of the myofilaments actin and myosin, the crossbridge formation, power strokes, and sustainability of the contraction itself.

A second and equally important property of skeletal muscle is the ability to return to an original shape after a contraction. This is called elasticity. Imagine an elastic band being stretched; after the stretch phase it returns to its original shape.

The ability to understand muscle activation and contraction provides a useful platform to examine whether muscles and soft tissues are functionally effective. Muscle testing enables the examiner to assess activation patterns together with the muscles' force production through either a static (fixed joint position) or dynamic (through a range of motion – ROM) contraction.

Muscle testing can range from a gentle hold to assess firing and activation, through to a resistive force being applied in the counter-direction to the muscle action. This text will consider different muscle test formats to illustrate the principles, instructions, positioning of client, and test directions, so that a greater appreciation for how testing is used can be developed. The terms "examiner" and "practitioner" have been used interchangeably throughout to highlight the different user populations of this text.

Manual muscle tests

This group of tests includes any strength test evaluation where the examiner applies resistance. This is appropriate for on-site and acute evaluations as no equipment is required apart from the examiner. Kisner and Colby (2002) further suggest that tests enable the examiner to control and adjust the resistance being applied in response to the client's efforts. Resistance can further be altered through the ROM (range of motion) to allow the client to achieve maximal effort throughout the test. A potential disadvantage to these tests is that all findings rely on subjective information and the examiner's ability to discern effective contraction from possible dysfunction. The examiner's own strength, posture, and morphology could negatively impact test findings.

Isometric break tests

Isometric break tests (Table 2) are relatively quick and efficient. They are performed in a neutral and midrange joint position. This position limits the stress being applied to the joint and could further reduce interference from non-contractile joint structures. For these tests it is important to instruct the client to hold the position, whilst the examiner supports and stabilizes the proximal segment, attempting to move the joint or "break" the position by applying a matching resistance to the distal segment. This resistive force is opposite but equal to the client's effort. To further confirm a strength test finding, it may be useful to stretch the muscle in the direction opposite to its motion. If one has a positive result of pain and some weakness from leg extensors, one may also note pain when stretching the leg extensors.

When grading a break test, it is important to grade the muscle according to the maximum resistance against which it holds. Table 3 contains an isometric grading scale that can be used to document findings.

Table 2	Isometric break tests
Strong and pain free	Indicates a normal response
Strong and painful	Potentially indicates a lesion in the musculotendinous junction or muscle. This is more common in acute injuries
Weak and pain free	Indicative of a nerve-related injury or musculotendinous rupture. It is important to note that contractile function could be lost without eliciting pain. This is dependent on rupture type and fiber damage
Weak and painful	Indicative of a serious injury that could range from bone trauma such as a fracture through to an unstable joint

Table 3	Break test grading scale*
Grade	Description
5	Maintains test position against gravity and maximal resistance
4	Maintains test position against gravity and moderate resistance
4–	Maintains test position against gravity and less than moderate resistance
3+	Maintains test position against gravity and minimal resistance
3	Maintains test position against gravity with no resistance

* Adapted from Clarkson (2000), cited in Shultz et al. (2016).

Graded manual muscle tests

These tests examine strength using applied resistance against gravity through a full or partial ROM. The tests provide more information than break tests as they examine and monitor muscle function throughout the ROM, not simply in the midrange, and better assess the individual muscle contributions. Muscles can be tested individually or within groups. Group tests do not always isolate contributions from individual muscles. Manual muscle tests could also provide more reliable information regarding the location and possible reason for muscle weakness and pain.

These tests are best performed by carefully positioning the client to be tested in such a way that the muscle being tested is easily isolated. The examiner stabilizes the proximal segment with one hand, whilst applying a resistance to the distal segment with the other. Anatomically translated this means stabilization is at the origin of the muscle with the resistance being applied at the insertion. The resistance should be applied in line with the orientation of the muscle fibers being tested. It is important to monitor compensation or substitution of muscle movements. This can easily be managed by careful client positioning and segmental stabilization.

Table 4 explains the criteria for gravity resisted muscle strength tests.

To be effective in manual muscle testing techniques it is important to identify and palpate muscles, as well as relate anatomy to muscle function and position.

Checklist for manual muscle testing techniques

- Provide clear communication and instruction to the client, including consent
- Identify origin, insertion, and motion of muscle or muscle group to be tested
- Observe and monitor possible compensatory movements and muscles, including breath-holding
- Position client for maximal support and stabilization
- Position self for best mechanical advantage and appropriate line of resistance
- Stabilize proximal segment
- Apply resistance to distal segment in direct line of pull with muscle function
- Complete the motion by monitoring any compensatory or substitution movements
- Reposition client to test with gravity minimized or eliminated if unable to complete the movement
- Use appropriate grading scale to document findings
- Record findings on clinical notes

Table 4 Criteria for gravity resisted muscle strength tests*

Numerical value	Word descriptor	Clinical description
5	Normal	Completes ROM against gravity and maximal resistance
4+		Completes ROM against gravity and against nearly maximal resistance
4	Good	Completes ROM against gravity and against moderate resistance
4–		Completes ROM against gravity and against minimal resistance >50% range
3+		Completes ROM against gravity and against minimal resistance <50% range
3	Fair	Completes ROM against gravity with no manual resistance
3–		Does not complete ROM against gravity but does complete more than half the range
2+		Initiates ROM against gravity or completes range with gravity minimized against slight resistance
2	Poor	Completes ROM with gravity minimized
2–		Unable to complete ROM with gravity minimized
1		Muscle contraction can be palpated but there is no joint motion
0	Zero	No palpable contraction or joint motion

* Adapted from Shultz et al. (2016).

In this section we have explored the isometric and isotonic muscle tests. In deciding which technique to use, a simple comparison between the techniques is needed (Table 5).

Kinesiology muscle testing

This method of muscle testing was introduced by Dr George Goodheart DC and used in applied kinesiology, and by chiropractors and other soft tissue practitioners (Cuthbert & Goodheart 2007). The client is passively placed into a position which brings the muscle's attachments (origin and insertion) closer together then asked to hold this position whilst the practitioner uses good, natural body movement, rocking their body slightly to place a small amount of pressure on the limb. If the muscle responds by activating contraction to match the light pressure, the muscle is deemed to be "strong." A "weak" test occurs when the client is unable to respond to this light movement and subsequent pressure.

Body movement is key to reliable testing. Practitioners should have excellent manual handling techniques and use swift and flowing movements to place the limb. Moving too slowly and ponderously will cause the client to recruit compensatory muscles.

Applied kinesiologists assign associations to certain muscles. They link muscles to acupuncture meridians and organs. This is widely seen in a branch of kinesiology called

Table 5	Comparison between isometric and isotonic muscle tests	
	Isometric	**Isotonic**
Advantages	Useful when moving a joint is difficult or contraindicated	Includes both concentric and eccentric strength components
	Requires minimal or no equipment	Enables examination of multiple muscles and joints
		Allows examination in closed-chain, weight bearing positions
		Provides a quantified metric for strength
Disadvantages	Measures strength of a specific joint position and not necessarily the function through a ROM	Limits maximal strength examination to the weakest point of the range
	Lacks objective strength measure	Allows stronger muscles to compensate or substitute for weaker muscles during multi-joint or muscle examination

Touch for Health. Some applied kinesiologists have recognized that certain emotional states can appear to weaken a muscle or groups of muscles. For completion, these associations have been listed within this book.

Palpation

Throughout this book, we explore palpation techniques. These are important in the location of soft tissue structures and ensure that testing of these structures is effective. Palpation is a difficult technique to master, and one which requires quality practice. Ideally, to palpate effectively, we need to see not with our eyes but with our hands and the pads of our fingers. Palpation is seeing through feeling and being able to identify different tissues and changes within tissue structure and tone. Biel and Dorn (2014), in their text *Trail Guide to the Human Body*, explain palpation by identifying three critical elements: "location," "becoming aware," and "assessment." The first two elements require a robust understanding of functional anatomy. Palpation requires skills of the hands through repetitive movements, coupled with an ability to listen, breathe calmly, and focus intensely on the structures being explored. Below are some useful hints to aid palpation skill development.

1. When you make contact, allow your fingers to be responsive and sensitive to the structures being explored. By using a double hand approach, i.e. one hand on top of another, you may be able to fine-tune the responsiveness and sensitivity within the palpating hand. Remember to be creative and use fingers to locate and palpate smaller structures, even using a supportive finger on the palpating finger.

2. Close your eyes to enable your awareness of the structures being palpated. Closing the eyes removes visual distractions and helps you to focus more intensely on locating different or specific structures.

3. Practice on your own body first. This is important in experiencing the technique and power of touch you may use on a client. By using your body as a practice guide, you become aware of pressures, comforts, discomforts, and structural changes. With consent, practice on other colleagues and listen to feedback.

4. Work smartly by researching the structures you wish to palpate prior to palpating. Keep the textbook open as you palpate. This will enable you to navigate the territory more effectively. Think of a road trip. If you research the route, identify places of interest, understand potential barriers, you will be more prepared and better enjoy the experience.

5. Be sensitive to your client's needs. When you begin palpating you may wish to explore deeper structures without fully locating access points to reach these structures. A good technique is to work slowly at first, by inviting the tissue into your hand. Carefully navigate borders and boundaries and communicate with your client to assess pressure and possibly pain outputs.

6. Familiarize yourself with the different palpation techniques such as gliding, strumming, rolling, and direct pressure. Follow structures and consider how they align or communicate with other structures.

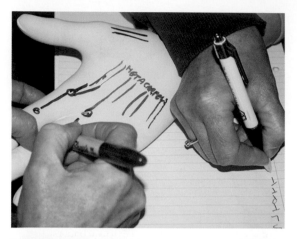

7. Use movement to help you identify and locate structural positions. Some structures are difficult to locate from a static position. By moving a limb, you can better access deeper structures. The application of a resistance force is useful in exposing structures and comparing bilateral alignments, shapes and configurations.

8. Practice feeling a grain of rice through a piece of paper. Then repeat, using a grain of sand. Use a mixture of cornstarch and water to make a thick paste. As you move your hand within the cornstarch mixture, you will note that smooth, sustained, flowing movements occur with ease, yet sharp, fast, and jabbing movements will be resisted by the cornstarch. Drop some small items in the cornstarch mixture and attempt to locate and identify them by touch.

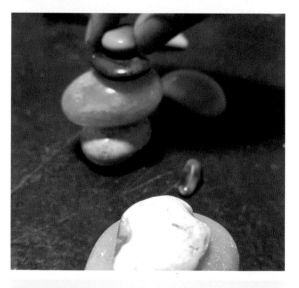

9. Use body painting to visualize key anatomical structures. Use skeletons or anatomical models to help refresh anatomical landmarks. You can use these as reference points for palpation within appropriate segments.

10. Improve palpation skills by practicing balancing pebbles one on another to make small towers. The dexterity needed to achieve balance will help palpation.

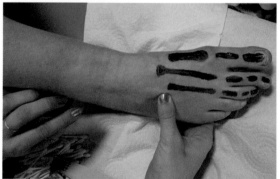

Improving palpation skills

In summary: Observe first, palpate second, and then use movement with palpation to locate muscles that lie deep to the surface.

Biotensegrity and fascia – the connective tissue system

When we begin to dissect the body and question the values of traditional models of anatomical learning, we soon realize that a more complicated and involved connective tissue system forms the framework that supports movement and enables complex movement patterns.

From embryonic development, we form a "meta-membrane" that ultimately weaves us together. This meta-membrane, or fascial web, provides the shape and form of our muscles and organs and ties together the structures that enable movement and function.

The underlying support stems from the fascial trains and slings that weave intricate webs and web patterns through the body, often connecting local, regional, and systemic components. Many anatomy teachers teach that the skeleton provides the strength for support within the body. If we remove the muscles, the skeleton is nothing more than a cluster of bones.

The biotensegrity geometry model explains that when stress is applied to the body, that stress is distributed rather than compressed. This begins to explain how local injuries can soon become global patterns of strain. The work of Tom Myers

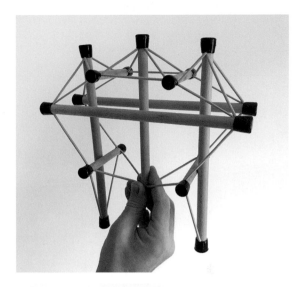

Biotensegrity representation of pelvis and legs

focuses on identifying and defining the fascial trains within the body to show how strain patterns are distributed within and throughout the connective tissue system via biotensegrity (Myers 2014).

The implications of fascia as a tensional network and framework within the body means that we must consider soft tissues when we perform muscle tests; a muscle can only work if the fascia surrounding and within it is under the correct tension.

How to use this book

Learning points

As the title of the book suggests, this is a concise guide which has been developed to enable students and practitioners to quickly access information by refreshing musculoskeletal anatomy and practically

Guide

This manual has been created to enable the reader to easily identify relevant information and facts and then learn or revise key muscle tests. The text layout is designed to consolidate learning by providing section headings, information and illustrations. Each section is separated by a line. Each chapter concludes with a QR code that links to a video which demonstrates the tests described, in a practical manner.

This section provides an anatomical overview and orientation of the muscle with its associated action, arterial and nerve supplies. Use this section to refresh, revise or learn the muscular anatomy.

Muscle Testing – TORSO AND TRUNK

PECTORALIS MAJOR (clavicular and sternal portions)

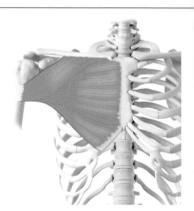

Origin
Upper fibers – **medial half of the clavicle**
Middle fibers – **anterolateral portion of the sternum**
Lower fibers – **costal cartilage of ribs 1–6**

Insertion
Lateral lip of bicipital groove of the humerus (crest of greater tubercle)

Action
All fibers:
Adduction and internal rotation of glenohumeral joint
Assists in elevation of thorax during forced inspiration (when the arm is fixed)
Upper fibers (clavicular portion):
Assists in horizontal adduction of glenohumeral joint
Flexion of shoulder at glenohumeral joint

Nerve supply
Medial and lateral pectoral nerve
C5–8, T1

Arterial supply
From thoracoabdominal trunk

The clinical facts section provides useful facts and information relevant to the muscle. This section focuses on clinical assessment and structural alignments.

Clinical facts
Works synergistically with latissimus dorsi, subscapularis, and teres major for adduction and internal rotation, and with the anterior fibers of the deltoid and coracobrachialis for flexion. The muscle can have multiple attachments on the ribs and sternum, so is an antagonist to itself. Considered an important respiratory muscle because of its attachments on or along the thoracic wall. The clavicular fibers tend to insert more distally, whereas the costo-sternal fibers insert proximally.
Aids shoulder flexion up to 60°. Pectoralis major is a powerful horizontal adductor and used to stabilize the torso during exercises such as push-ups, bench press, throwing and punching movements. Over-development of the muscles may negatively impact shoulder posture and result in a more round-shouldered appearance. Unilateral absence of the muscle indicates a congenital disorder called Poland syndrome which affects males more than females.

Palpation

1. Client is either supine, side lying or seated, with shoulder (GHJ) forward flexed to 90°.

2. Place palpating fingers over the muscle fibers, carefully feeling the region you wish to examine. Remember to follow the fiber patterns.

3. To fully palpate the contraction of the muscle fibers, ask the client to move their arm across their chest (horizontal adduction) whilst a counter resistance force is applied by the examiner.

4. Note the contraction within the muscle tissue.

5. A more sensitive palpatory technique involves the examiner pinching, or firmly gripping the anterior axillary fold, whilst the client's arm is in forward flexion.

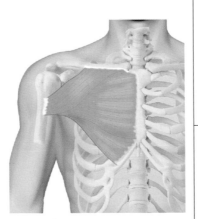

A key to successful muscle testing is learning to palpate and locate the muscle. This section is designed to provide guidance and signposting for locating the muscle and its associated attachment structures, by carefully understanding both the surface and deeper anatomical orientations.

Manual muscle test

Position Supine
For this muscle, the test is delivered in 2 parts, one for the sternal head, the other for the clavicular one.
Sternal head (A)
Supine, with shoulder (glenohumeral joint) flexed to 90°, with arm fully internally rotated.
Clavicular head (B)
Supine, with shoulder (GHJ) flexed to 90°, with arm internally rotated to roughly 45°

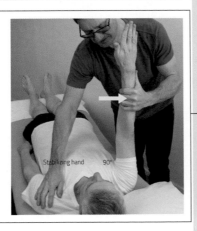

Stabilizing hand 90°

This section is designed carefully to guide the user through a series of considerations; patient positioning, force generation and stabilization techniques to ensure effective and accurate testing of muscles. The muscle tests are further divided into graded, manual, and kinesiological. The section concludes with a video code for an instructional recording of the techniques described in the text.

Pectoralis major

applying the techniques illustrated. With over 60 muscles, each muscle detailed in the book provides the reader with an overview of the origin, insertion, muscle fiber arrangements, nerve and blood supply and action. This is important in considering different muscle tests. Each muscle test is described through photographs, videos, and annotation. It is important to note – as the title of the book implies – that only selected muscles have been included. The idea is to relate more popular and common muscle tests to muscular function.

When using this text, consider the following learning points to help consolidate your knowledge and practical skills.

1. Anatomy – begin by using a skeleton or an anatomical model to help visualize and identify structural location, attachments, congruency, and depth of structure. This may enable you to develop an appreciation for palpation and access of musculoskeletal structures. Simply knowing a muscle's location, without considering associated structures, neurovascular pathways, and other relational structures, may be insufficient to enable palpation and testing of the structure.

2. Function – it is important to carefully consider full function of the muscle being assessed and tested. In your learning or revision of the neuromuscular system, consider all movements and accessory movement patterns that are common to the muscle/s being studied. This will enable a greater recognition of client positioning and test execution. Consider synergists, agonists and antagonists, and the effect of a muscle when it is eccentrically loaded.

3. Individual versus group testing – muscle testing may appear complex at times and multiple approaches regarding testing position and reliability may need to be considered. One such approach could pertain to whether it is more effective to test a group of muscles, e.g. flexors of the forearm, or isolated individual muscles. To discern which is best, one needs to understand the value and purpose of muscle testing. Muscle tests are used during musculoskeletal assessments but can equally be useful in treatment strategies where strength, or lack thereof, becomes a key clinical marker. In deciding how to approach muscle testing and which test/s to use, consider the questions listed in the box on the next page.

Questions to ask yourself

1. What does the test reveal?
2. What does the test fail to reveal?
3. Has the test been executed correctly?
4. Are the client instructions clear and unambiguous?
5. Is the client positioned correctly?
6. Should I use muscle tests if the client reports painful responses to the test?
7. When is the best time to use or implement muscle testing in the musculoskeletal assessment process?
8. How conclusive is the test in enabling me to justify my thinking/findings and proposed treatment strategies?
9. Have I related my anatomical understanding to the test findings?
10. Have I considered anatomical variations in neuromuscular tissue?
11. What do the test findings reveal in relation to neurovascular orientation?
12. Are there other tests that can be used to confirm or reject my current findings?
13. Have incongruencies and/or specificity factors been accounted for?
14. What is the client telling me about the experience of the test?
15. Do I use the information received from clients and the tests to make informed choices about healthcare and client management?

References

Barral J (2008) *Understanding the messages of your body*, Berkeley, CA: North Atlantic Books.

Biel A and Dorn R (2014) *Trail guide to the human body*, Boulder, CO: Books of Discovery.

Clarkson HM (2000) *Musculoskeletal assessment, joint range of motion and manual muscle strength*, 2nd edn, London: Lippincott Williams and Wilkins.

Cuthbert SC and Goodheart GJ (2007) On the reliability and validity of manual muscle testing: A literature review. *Chiropractic and Manual Therapies* 15:4. https://doi.org/10.1186/1746-1340-15-4

Kisner C and Colby LA (2002) *Therapeutic exercise: Foundations and techniques*, 5th edn, Philadelphia: FA Davis Co.

Myers T (2014) *Anatomy trains: Myofascial meridians for manual and movement therapists*, New York: Churchill Livingstone, Elsevier.

Shultz SJ, Houglum PA and Perrin DH (2016) *Examination of musculoskeletal injuries*, 4th edn, Champaign, IL: Human Kinetics.

Thie J (1973) *Touch for Health*, Camarillo, CA: De Vorss & Co.

Vizniak NA (2012) *Muscle manual*, Canada: Professional Health Systems Inc.

Walther D (2000) *Applied kinesiology (synopsis)*, 2nd edn, USA: Systems DC.

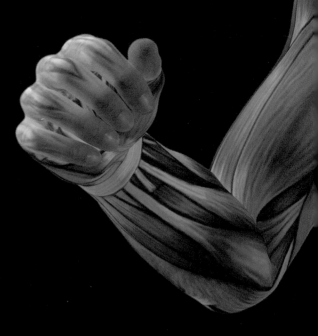

Section

2

MUSCLE TESTS BY REGION

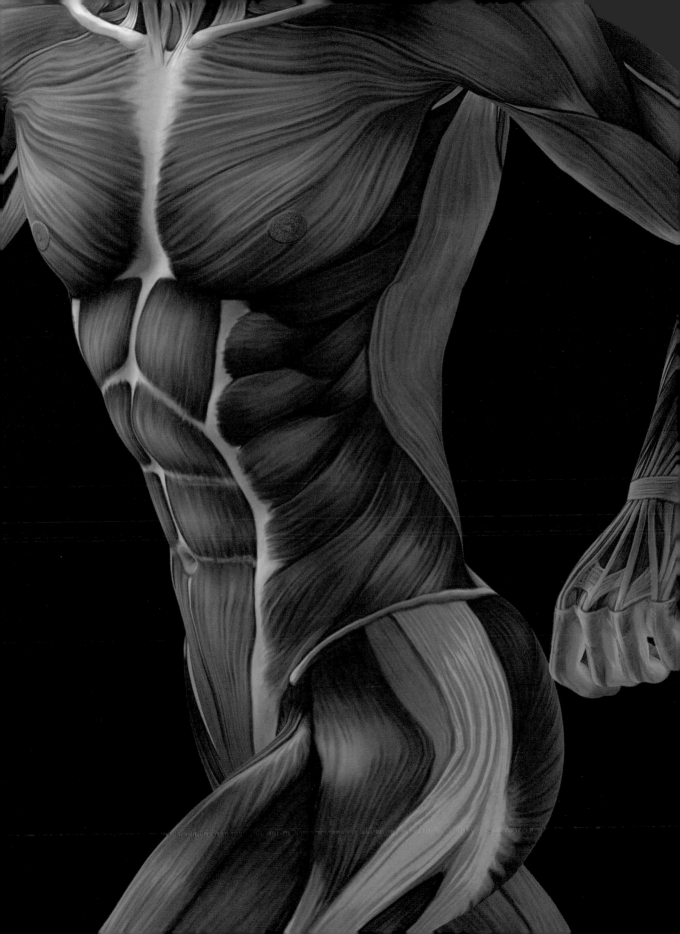

STERNOCLEIDOMASTOID (SCM)

The name of this muscle provides important attachment information: sterno = sternum, cleido = clavicle, mastoid = mastoid process of the temporal bone.

Origin

Sternal head – manubrium of sternum
Clavicular head – medial clavicle

Insertion

Mastoid process of temporal bone

Action

Rotation of head and neck to the contralateral side
Lateral flexion of head and neck to the ipsilateral side
Bilaterally the muscle aids in forward flexion of the neck and assists elevation of the ribs during inhalation
Helps to control neck extension by eccentrically loading the sternocleidomastoid

Nerve supply

Spinal accessory nerve (CN XI), C2–C3

Arterial supply

Occipital artery
Superior thyroid artery

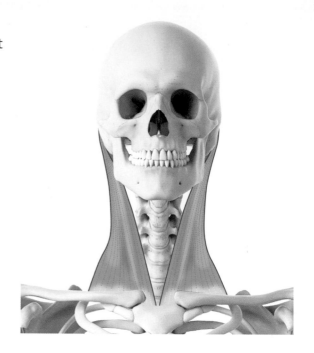

Clinical facts

Upper fibers of sternocleidomastoid may blend with the posterior lateral edge of the trapezius.

Based on the attachment points on the sternum and clavicle, some anatomists argue that an associated function of the muscle is the elevation of the anterior aspect of the ribcage, thereby describing it, in part, as an accessory respiratory muscle.

The position of sternocleidomastoid, especially its medial border, makes it susceptible to vascular traumas. The medial aspect lies close to the carotid arteries and sinus. Palpation of sternocleidomastoid requires careful consideration as increased pressure over the carotid sinus and artery could lead to a drop in blood pressure and a possible bout of unconsciousness.

Excessive hyperextension and/or flexion, e.g. whiplash trauma, could lead to tears within sternocleidomastoid.

Palpation

1. Client is seated or supine with the head rotated to one side. With this position, a visual examination will reveal the borders of the muscle.

2. Place palpating fingers over the muscle fibers and instruct the client to flex or rotate their head to one side. Caution should be exercised when palpating as increased pressure could impede vascular function.

3. Note the contraction within the muscle tissue.

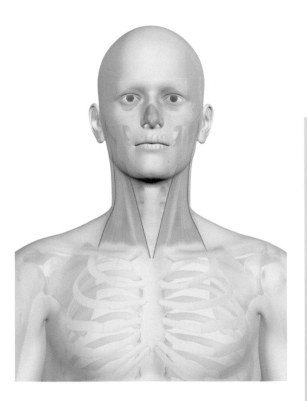

Manual muscle test

Position

Supine with neck flexed and slightly rotated to contralateral side.

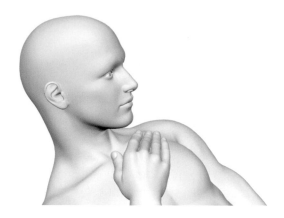

Test

Examiner applies a resistance force posteriorly and laterally by placing their hand over the lateral aspect of the frontal bone. It is important to follow the anatomical landmarks of sternocleidomastoid identified during palpation.

Use an appropriate grading scale to record the findings. Remember to test through the range.

A midrange test can be used to assess isometric strength, wherein the client is instructed to hold the position without a resistant force being applied by the examiner.

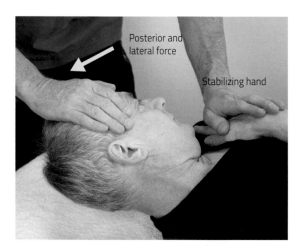

Posterior and lateral force

Stabilizing hand

Stabilization

Stabilization occurs over the sternum. It is good practice to ask the client to place their free hand over their own chest. The examiner then places their hand on top of the client's hand.

Kinesiology muscle test

Position

Supine. Lift the head into slight flexion and contralateral rotation, as if bringing the ear toward the shoulder, thus bringing attachments of sternocleidomastoid closer together.

Test

Client is instructed to hold this position. Examiner rocks their own body slightly, exerting a light force downward on the contralateral frontal bone, as if to return the head to the couch.

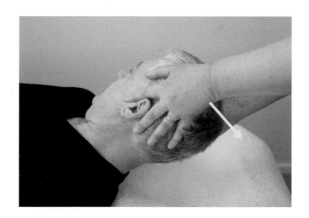

Stabilization

Examiner supports head movement by cupping the other side of the head, preventing any injury should sternocleidomastoid be too weak to hold in position.

Kinesiological associations

Organ: Stomach, sinuses, and lymphatic system
Acupuncture meridian: Stomach
Emotion: Worry and emotional stress

Video: Sternocleidomastoid (SCM)

SCALENES (anterior, middle, and posterior)

Origin

Anterior scalene
Transverse processes of 3rd, 4th, 5th, and 6th cervical vertebrae
Middle scalene
Transverse processes of 2nd, 3rd, 4th, 5th, 6th, and 7th cervical vertebrae
Posterior scalene
Transverse processes of 5th, 6th, and 7th cervical vertebrae

Insertion

Anterior scalene
Scalene tubercle of the 1st rib
Middle scalene
2nd rib
Posterior scalene
2nd rib

Action

Anterior scalene
Flexion and ipsilateral flexion of the neck
Elevation of 1st rib
Acts as a weak contralateral rotator of the neck when the neck is stabilized
Helps to control extension of the neck when eccentrically loaded
Middle scalene
Flexion and ipsilateral flexion of the neck
Helps to control extension of the neck when eccentrically loaded
Elevation of 2nd rib when the neck is stabilized

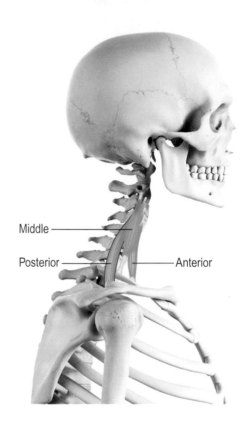

Posterior scalene
Flexion and ipsilateral flexion of neck
Helps to control extension of the neck when eccentrically loaded
Elevation of 2nd rib when the neck is stabilized

Nerve supply

Anterior scalene
Spinal nerves C3, C4, C5, C6

Middle scalene
Spinal nerves C6, C7, C8
Posterior scalene
Spinal nerves C6, C7, C8

Arterial supply

Anterior, middle, and posterior scalene
Inferior thyroid artery

Clinical facts

Anterior, middle, and posterior scalenes work synergistically with each other. The scalene group are an accessory or supportive muscle in respiration. Scalenes are used when taking a deep breath into the upper chest and to hold a phone between ear and shoulder. Scalenes are more likely to become hypertonic (too tight) than hypotonic

(too weak). The large branches of brachial plexus and subclavian artery pass through a small gap between the anterior and middle scalenes. These can become impinged if the scalenes are hypertonic, causing pain or numbness and pins and needles.
Some anatomists note that the posterior scalenes may occasionally attach to the lateral border of the 3rd rib.

Palpation

VERY IMPORTANT: Due to the neurovascular bundles that are present near the anatomical location of the scalenes, palpation should proceed with extreme caution to avoid disruption of or potential harm to the underlying neurovascularity.

Anterior and middle scalenes

1. Client is usually seated or supine.
2. Carefully rotate the client's head to the contralateral side being palpated and make sure you move sternocleidomastoid (SCM) out of the way.

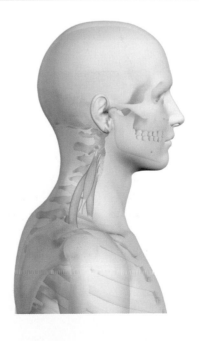

3. Place palpating fingers lateral to the SCM and superiorly to the medial aspect of the clavicle.

4. To fully expose and palpate the muscle belly, the client should be instructed to inhale deeply.

5. Palpation of the clavicle is key as the anterior and middle scalenes can further be palpated inferiorly behind the medial aspect of the clavicle.

6. Remember the scalenes function as a group so medial to the middle scalenes are the anterior fibers of the scalenes.

Posterior scalene

1. Client is usually seated or supine.

2. Palpate middle fibers and the levator scapulae, ensuring you place palpating fingers between these muscles.

3. To fully expose and palpate the muscle belly, the client should be instructed to inhale deeply.

4. To functionally locate and palpate the posterior fibers of the scalenes, instruct the client to elevate and depress the scapula alternately.

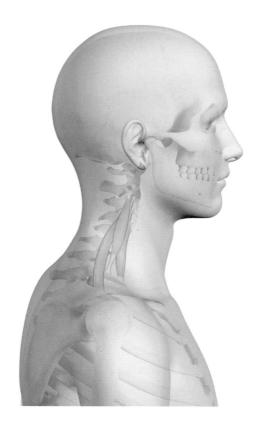

Manual muscle test

Position

Supine with the head elevated and rotated to the contralateral side being tested; with the hands folded behind the head.

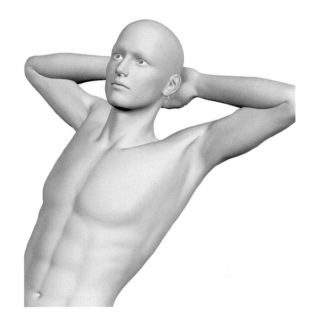

Test

Client is requested to inhale deeply and then flex their head to their chest against the practitioner's mild (25%) resistance.

Stabilization

Practitioner stands at the head of the table with the fingers of their hand stabilizing the client's forehead.

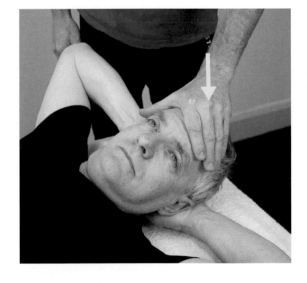

Kinesiology muscle test

Position

Performed supine. Bend the elbows and place the client's hands level with their ears. Slightly flex the head forward and rotate it 10° away from the side being tested.

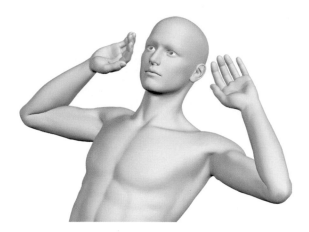

Test

Ask the client to maintain this position. Practitioner places the side of the hand on client's forehead rather than using the whole hand. Practitioner slightly rocks their own body, exerting a light pressure on the center of the forehead; direction is directly down toward the couch (not in line with the rotation of the client's head).

Stabilization

Client isolates the scalenes as much as possible by bringing the arms and hands up. Watch for recruitment; if scalenes are weak, client may attempt to further rotate or laterally tilt the head to recruit other muscles to help, including breath-holding.

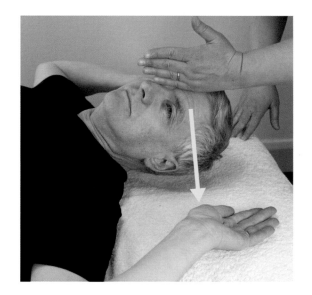

Kinesiological associations

Organ: Stomach, sinuses
Acupuncture meridian: Stomach
Emotion: Worry

Video: Scalene group

SPLENIUS CAPITIS

Origin
Spinous processes of C3–T4 vertebrae and inferior portion of the nuchal line

Insertion
Mastoid process of temporal bone and superior portion of nuchal line

Action
Unilateral
Ipsilateral rotation and lateral flexion of head and neck
Bilateral
Extension of head and neck
Helps to control neck flexion when eccentrically loaded

Nerve supply
Cervical spinal nerves C2, C3, C4, C5, C6

Arterial supply
Occipital artery

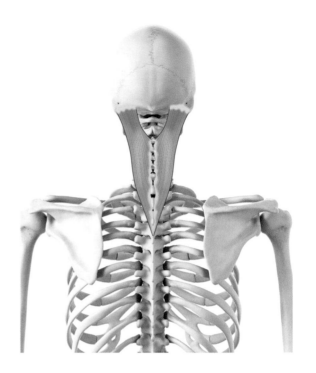

Clinical facts
Works synergistically with the trapezius, semispinalis, scalenes, and longus capitis. Forms a V shape on the posterior aspect of the neck.
Splenius capitis may only form attachments from T3 and above.
Painful splenius capitis and splenius cervicis may mimic migraine, causing severe head and neck pain, particularly around the eye. This can be triggered by looking upward for long periods, such as when painting a ceiling. It is also triggered by maintaining a head tilt for long periods, such as listening on a phone, poor office posture, or in an accident causing whiplash.

Palpation

1. The splenius muscles are deep to trapezius therefore palpation should be performed carefully using pads of the fingers.
2. Client is placed prone, with palpating hand following the directions of the muscle fibers.
3. The client should be instructed to extend their head and neck.

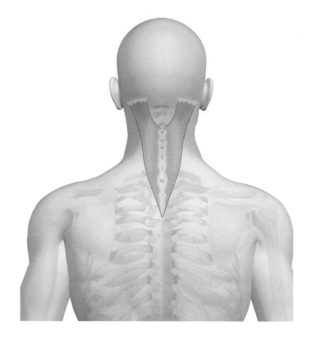

Manual muscle test

Position

Prone, head laterally flexed, rotated and slightly extended to the ipsilateral side.

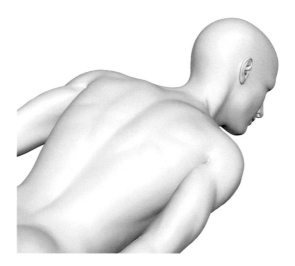

Test

Practitioner applies a strong resistance (about 75%) toward forward flexion and roughly 25% toward opposite side lateral flexion. This should always be done in the direction of the muscle fibers.

Stabilization

A stabilizing hand is placed firmly on the upper portion of the thoracic spine.

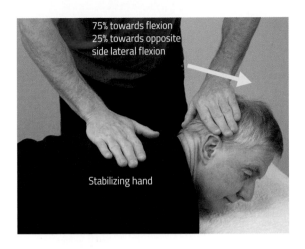

75% towards flexion
25% towards opposite
side lateral flexion

Stabilizing hand

Kinesiology muscle test

Position

Unilaterally
Prone, lift the head into neck extension, and rotate the head slightly to one side.
Bilaterally
Prone, lift the head into neck extension.

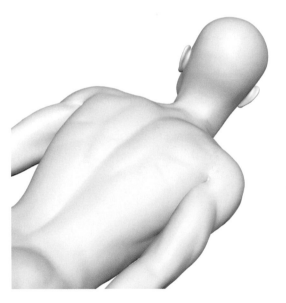

Test

Unilaterally and bilaterally
Ask client to hold the position. Practitioner places a hand on the posterior surface of the client's head, and rocks their own body slightly, exerting a light pressure on the head as if to press the head down toward the couch.

Stabilization

Support the head carefully when testing to prevent head hitting the couch if these muscles are weak.

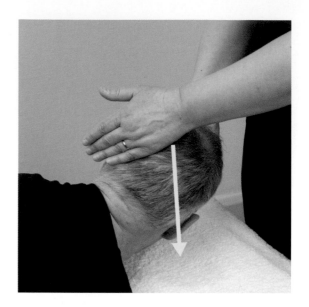

Kinesiological associations

Organ: Cervical and lumbar spine, sacroiliac joint, stomach, sinuses
Acupuncture meridian: Stomach
Emotion: Worry

Video: Splenius capitis

LEVATOR SCAPULAE

Origin
Transverse processes of C1 to C4 vertebrae

Insertion
Superior medial border of scapula

Action
Elevation of the scapula coupled with extension and lateral flexion of the neck
Helps to control neck extension on the contralateral side and scapula abduction in the later stage when eccentrically loaded

Nerve supply
Cervical and dorsal scapular nerve
C3, C4, C5

Arterial supply
Dorsal scapular artery

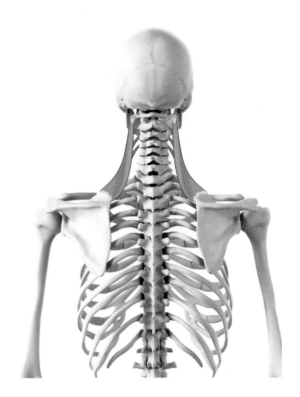

Clinical facts

Works synergistically with the upper fibers of trapezius.

It is relatively common for the cervical vertebra attachments to vary (e.g. C1–C3). Some levator scapulae fibers may attach to occipital bone, mastoid process of temporal bone, or 1st to 2nd ribs.

Levator scapulae fibers are known to merge with those of the trapezius, serratus anterior, and scalenes.

Muscle tension is often reported in the mid region of the muscle due to the anatomical positioning resulting in a spiral adaptation. Clinicians may mistake this for myofascial trigger points.

Damage to the muscle may result in sensory disturbances such as numbness and paresthesia.

Palpation

1. Client may be seated or prone with the forearm comfortably positioned over the lower back with palm facing upward. In this position, the fibers of the levator scapulae are more accessible as the trapezius is relaxed.

2. The palpating hand is then placed superiorly to the angle of the scapula.

3. To best locate the belly of levator scapulae, the client can elevate and then depress their scapula on the side being palpated.

4. Palpate along the muscle fibers as levator scapulae extends to the lateral aspect of the neck.

5. Remember levator scapulae is deep to the trapezius so practice palpation with eyes closed to feel through muscle tissue.

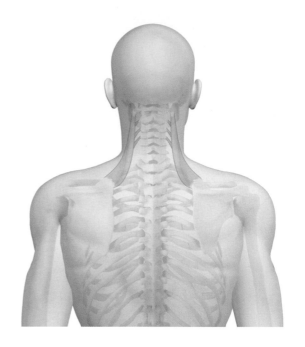

Manual muscle test

Position

Seated, with head laterally flexed, rotated and slightly extended to the ipsilateral side.

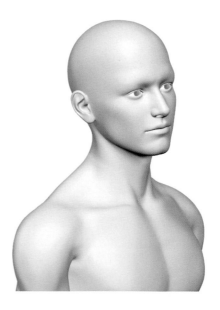

Test

Practitioner applies a strong (about 75%) resistance toward opposite lateral flexion and roughly 25% inferiorly toward scapula. This should always be done in the direction of the muscle fibers.

Stabilization

Stabilizing hand is placed firmly on the ipsilateral shoulder.

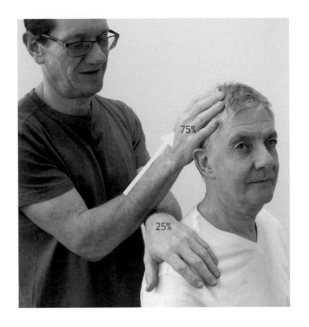

Kinesiology muscle test

Position

Seated or supine. Flex the elbow and maximally drop the shoulder by giving shoulder traction down toward hip until engagement of the neck and head is observed. Adduct and slightly extend the humerus. There should be minimal lumbar side bending.

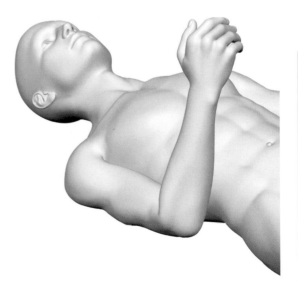

Test

Client is instructed to hold this position. Practitioner rocks their own body slightly, exerting a light pull on the medial elbow toward abduction. Watch for inferior rotation of the superior angle of scapula rather than feeling a lock in the test. It is easy to be too heavy-handed.

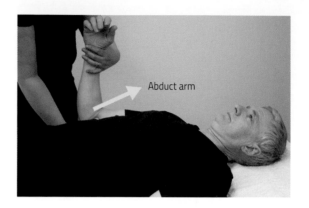

Abduct arm

Stabilization

Stabilize the test by supporting the ipsilateral shoulder to encourage it to be pulled downward.

Kinesiological associations

Organ: Lung and parathyroid
Acupuncture meridian: Lung
Emotion: Grief and stress

Video: Levator scapulae

TRAPEZIUS (upper fibers)

Origin

Trapezius muscles have multiple origins which include:
External occipital protuberance
Medial superior nuchal line and nuchal ligament
Spinous processes C7–T12
Upper fibers are classed as originating from external occipital protuberance and medial superior nuchal line and nuchal ligament.

Insertion

Trapezius muscles have multiple insertions, which include: lateral third of clavicle, acromion, and spine of scapula
Insertion of upper fibers at clavicle may extend from lateral third to mid clavicle just superior to deltoid origin. It may also blend with posterior and lateral edge of sternocleidomastoid

Action

Elevation and retraction of scapula, culminating in adduction of the scapula
Upward rotation of the scapula which is caused by co-contraction of the upper and lower fibers
Upper fibers enable the last 60° of glenohumeral flexion and abduction
Fibers of upper trapezius act unilaterally to laterally flex the head and bilaterally to assist in head extension
Further stabilization of the scapula during elevated arm movements

Nerve supply

Spinal accessory nerve (CN XI), C2–C4

Arterial supply

Transverse cervical and dorsal scapular arteries

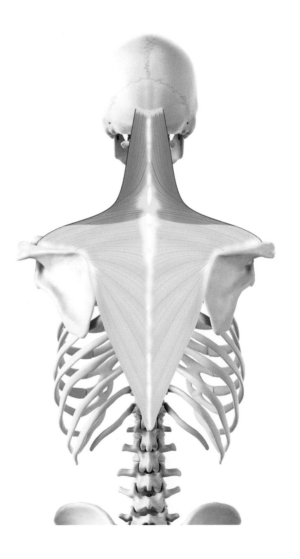

Clinical facts

The trapezius muscle is typically divided into three functional parts: upper, middle, and lower fibers. It acts within a composite contraction of these fibers to influence, stabilize, and enhance scapula, thoracic, and shoulder movements.

Embryologically, upper trapezius develops from the same branch of mesoderm as sternocleidomastoid. Both upper trapezius and sternocleidomastoid muscles have cranial nerve innervation (CN XI – spinal accessory nerve).

Greater occipital nerve traverses the upper fibers of trapezius. Tightness and/or physical trauma, chronic stress, or anxiety could result in compression of greater occipital nerve, leading to headaches, dizziness, and visual interruptions.

Damage to upper trapezius fibers will lead to a drooped posture of the ipsilateral shoulder resulting in weakness through the last 60° of glenohumeral abduction.

Palpation

1. Performed prone.
2. Place palpating hand over the upper trapezius fibers by carefully considering origin and insertional points.
3. Ask client to raise their arm/shoulder against some resistance which can be applied through the non-palpating hand.
4. To more thoroughly palpate upper trapezius fibers, ask client to slightly extend the head and neck.

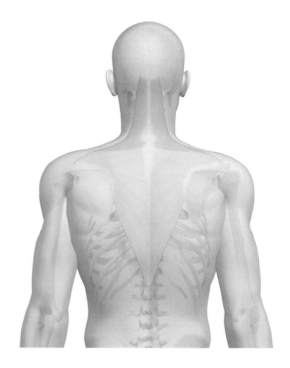

Manual muscle testing

Position

Seated or prone. If seated, it is important to ensure that the head is laterally flexed toward, rotated away and slightly extended from the side being tested.

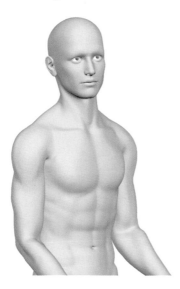 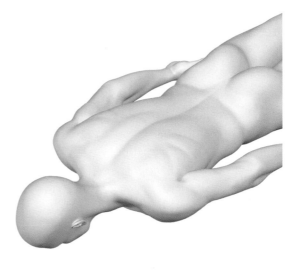

Test

The examiner places one hand on the lateral side of the head with the other hand crossed over and placed on shoulder. Hands are in a crossed position to prevent use of too much force. Examiner applies a resistance force of about 75% toward opposite lateral flexion of the head. A further 25% of force is applied downward over glenohumeral joint. Remember: upper trapezius fibers can also be tested bilaterally by resisting shoulder elevation (likened to the test for levator scapulae).

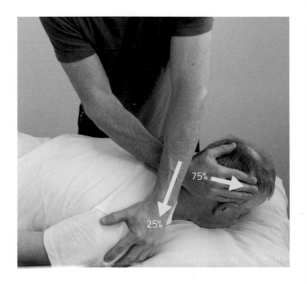

Use an appropriate grading scale to record the findings. Remember to test through the range.
A midrange test can be used to assess isometric strength, wherein the client is instructed to hold the position without a resistant force being applied by the examiner.

Stabilization

Stabilization occurs over the ipsilateral shoulder using a "crossed arms" posture.

Kinesiology muscle test

Position

Prone
Abduct straight arm 45° and slightly extend arm back 30°, thus bringing scapula into adduction and bringing upper trapezius attachments closer together. Slightly externally rotate humerus so thumb is pointing toward the floor.

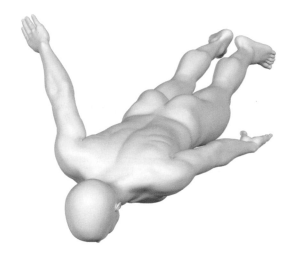

Seated
Laterally flex head toward shoulder whilst elevating shoulder to meet head.

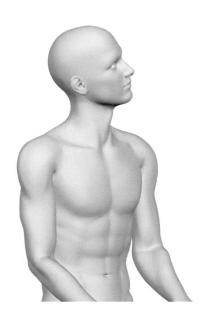

Test

Prone

Client is instructed to hold the position of arm whilst examiner rocks their own body, slightly exerting a light force downward on the distal forearm toward flexion, as if to bring the arm toward the floor.

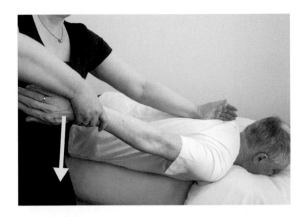

Seated

Client is instructed to hold this position. Examiner crosses their arms and presses lightly on both shoulder and lateral side of head, as if to move both shoulder and head apart.

Warning: this method can induce painful cramping in upper trapezius so should be avoided if hypertonic upper trapezius is suspected.

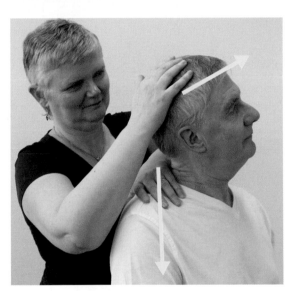

Stabilization

Prone

Examiner stabilizes the movement by placing the edge of their supporting hand lightly on lower ribs.

Seated

Stabilization occurs over the ipsilateral shoulder using a "crossed arms" posture.

Kinesiological associations

Organ: Kidney, ears and eyes
Acupuncture meridian: Kidney
Emotion: Fear and emotional stress

Video: Trapezius (upper fibers)

TRAPEZIUS (middle fibers)

Origin

Trapezius muscles have multiple origins which include:
External occipital protuberance
Medial superior nuchal line and nuchal ligament
Spinous processes C7–T12
Middle trapezius fibers are classed as originating from C7 to upper thoracic vertebrae (approximately at T3)

Insertion

Trapezius muscles have multiple insertions which include: lateral third of clavicle, acromion, and spine of scapula
Insertion of middle trapezius fibers may extend to medial edge of acromion and posterior border of spine of scapula

Action

Elevation and retraction of scapula – culminating in adduction of the scapula
Stabilization of scapula during arm movements
Helps to control scapula abduction when eccentrically loaded

Nerve supply

Spinal accessory nerve (CN X1)
Ventral rami C2–C4

Arterial supply

Transverse cervical and dorsal scapular arteries

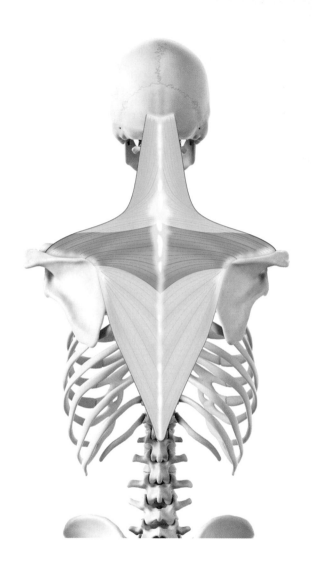

Clinical facts

Trapezius is clinically divided into three distinct fibers (upper, middle, and lower), and is most active during the last 50–60° of shoulder flexion and abduction. Works synergistically with levator scapulae for elevation, rhomboids for retraction of the scapula, and latissimus dorsi for shoulder (GHJ) depression.

Postural malalignments such as an anterior head carriage with rounded shoulders may result in fatigue of the trapezius leading to postural fatigue syndrome.
If the trapezius is paralyzed, the ipsilateral shoulder will drop, and the individual will struggle with shoulder abduction past 60°.

Palpation

1. Prone.
2. Place palpating fingers over middle fibers of trapezius.
3. Instruct the client to abduct their shoulder (GHJ) to 90°. A mild over-pressure could be applied to the abducted arm.
4. Note the contraction within the muscle tissue. Remember that during shoulder abduction there is a natural upward rotation of the scapula which involves co-contraction of the upper and lower fibers.

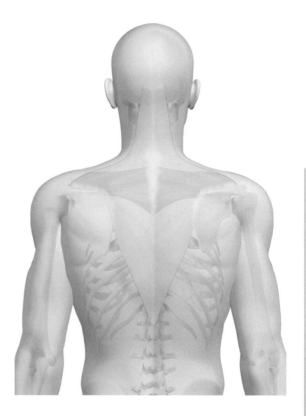

Manual muscle test

Position

Prone. Shoulder is abducted to 90° and humerus is externally rotated.

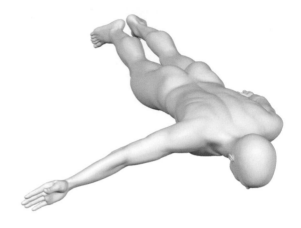

Test

Examiner applies a resistance force downward toward the floor in a horizontal adducted position.

Use an appropriate grading scale to record the findings. Remember to test through the range.

A midrange test can be used to assess isometric strength, wherein the client is instructed to hold the position without a resistance force being applied by the examiner.

Stabilization

Examiner can place a stabilizing arm over the contralateral scapula.

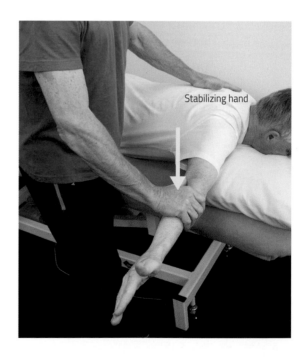

Stabilizing hand

Kinesiology muscle test

Position

Prone, with arm abducted to 90° and externally rotated as far as is comfortable for the client, ideally with thumb pointing toward ceiling.

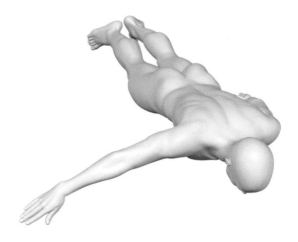

Test

Client is instructed to hold the position of arm whilst examiner rocks their own body slightly, exerting a light force downward on the distal forearm toward flexion, as if to bring the arm toward the floor.

Test is deemed to be strong by observing for contraction of middle trapezius fibers invoking adduction of scapula toward the vertebral column. If no adduction of scapula occurs, the test is weak. Do not rely on the client's ability to maintain arm position. Watch for recruitment of other muscles, including breath-holding.

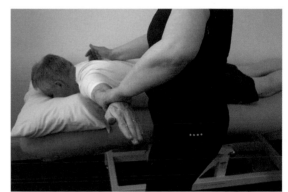

Stabilization

Examiner can stabilize by placing the edge of the hand on the lower ribs on the contralateral side.

Kinesiological associations

Organ: Spleen
Acupuncture meridian. Spleen pancreas
Emotion: Worry, tiredness

Video: Trapezius (middle fibers)

TRAPEZIUS (lower fibers)

Origin

Trapezius muscles have multiple origins which include:
External occipital protuberance
Medial superior nuchal line and nuchal ligament
Spinous processes C7–T12
Lower trapezius fibers are classed as originating from spinous processes of mid/lower thoracic vertebrae (around T4 to T12)

Insertion

Trapezius muscles have multiple insertions, which include: lateral third of clavicle, acromion, and spine of scapula
Insertion of lower trapezius fibers extend into an aponeurosis at medial portion of spine of scapula

Action

Elevation and retraction of scapula – culminating in adduction and upward rotation of the scapula
Gives inferior stabilization of scapula during arm movements

Nerve supply

Spinal accessory nerve (CN X1)
Ventral rami C2–C4

Arterial supply

Transverse cervical and dorsal scapular arteries

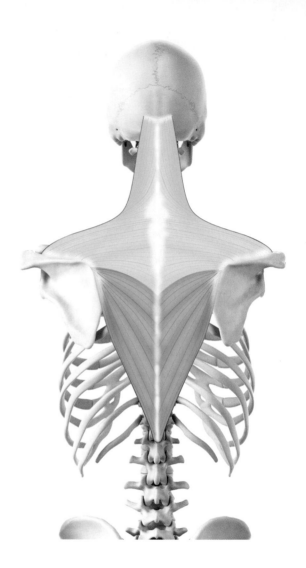

Clinical facts

Trapezius is clinically divided into three distinct fibers (upper, middle, and lower), and is most active during the last 50–60° of shoulder flexion and abduction. Works synergistically with levator scapulae for elevation, rhomboids for retraction of the scapula, and latissimus dorsi for shoulder (GHJ) depression.

Postural malalignments such as an anterior head carriage with rounded shoulders may result in fatigue of the trapezius leading to postural fatigue syndrome.
If the trapezius is paralyzed, the ipsilateral shoulder will drop, and the individual will struggle with shoulder abduction past 60°.

Palpation

1. Prone.
2. Place palpating fingers over lower fibers of trapezius.
3. Instruct the client to abduct their shoulder (GHJ) to 120°. A mild over-pressure could be applied to the abducted arm.
4. Note the contraction within the muscle tissue. Remember that during shoulder abduction there is a natural upward rotation of the scapula which involves co-contraction of the upper and lower fibers.

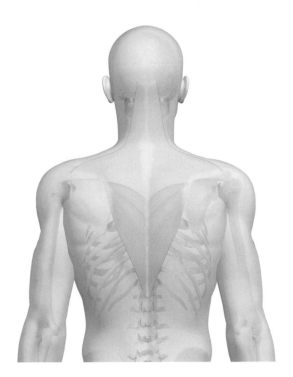

Manual muscle test

Position

Prone. Shoulder is abducted to 120° and humerus is externally rotated.

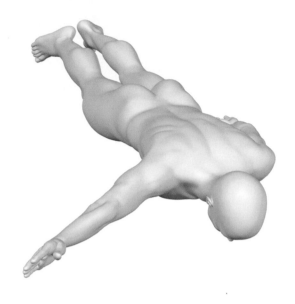

Test

Examiner applies a resistance force downward toward the floor in a horizontal adducted position.

Use an appropriate grading scale to record the findings. Remember to test through the range.

A midrange test can be used to assess isometric strength, wherein the client is instructed to hold the position without a resistant force being applied by the examiner.

Stabilization

Examiner can place a stabilizing arm over the contralateral scapula.

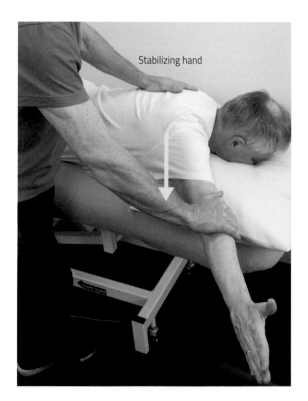

Stabilizing hand

Kinesiology muscle test

Position

Prone, with arm abducted to 120–150°, so arm is in line with the fibers of lower trapezius and externally rotated as far as is comfortable for the client, ideally with thumb pointing toward ceiling.

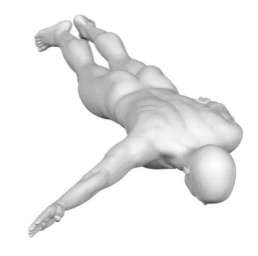

Test

Client is instructed to hold the position of arm whilst examiner rocks their own body slightly, exerting a light force downward on the distal forearm toward flexion, as if to bring the arm toward the floor.
Test is deemed to be strong by observing for contraction of lower trapezius fibers invoking adduction of scapula toward the vertebral column. If no adduction of scapula occurs, the test is weak. Do not rely on the client's ability to maintain arm position. Watch for recruitment of other muscles, including breath-holding and elbow flexion.

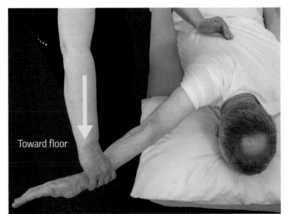

Toward floor

Stabilization

Examiner can stabilize by placing the edge of the hand on the lower ribs.

Kinesiological associations

Organ: Spleen
Acupuncture meridian: Spleen pancreas
Emotion: Worry, tiredness

Video: Trapezius (lower fibers)

SUPRASPINATUS

The rotator cuff group comprises the "SITS" muscles, namely the supraspinatus, infraspinatus, teres minor, and subscapularis. It is an important group of muscles that enables movement and stabilization of the glenohumeral joint (GHJ). This is an incredibly unstable joint and compromises stability for mobility, so requires functioning muscles surrounding the joint to maintain stability. Imagine a golf ball sitting on a tee, with the ball being almost double the size of the tee surface. This analogy describes the relationship between the larger humeral head (the golf ball), and the smaller and shallower glenoid fossa (the golf tee).

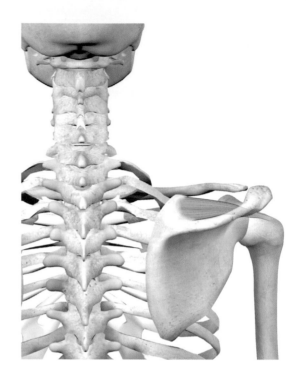

Origin

Supraspinous fossa of scapula

Insertion

Superior facet of greater tubercle of humerus

Action

Abduction of shoulder (glenohumeral joint) with slight flexion
Holds upper limb away from torso
Helps to control adduction with slight extension of shoulder during eccentric contraction

Nerve supply

Suprascapular nerve
C5, C6

Arterial supply

Suprascapular artery

Clinical facts

Works synergistically with the middle fibers of deltoid.

Only "rotator cuff" muscle that does not cause rotation at the shoulder.

Suprascapular nerve entrapment could negatively impact muscle action.

Excessive strain and trauma can, over time, cause tendonitis or tendinopathies which may be associated with calcific tendonitis.

It passes under the subacromial space and is protected by the subacromial bursa.

Irritation of the subacromial bursa can lead to bursitis.

After the age of 40, ruptures and tears of the supraspinatus tendon are more common.

Palpation

1. Client is either prone or seated.
2. Locate the acromion process and follow it medially and posteriorly. This will enable the palpation of the spine of the scapula.
3. Palpation is conducted superior to the spine of the scapula in line with the directions of the fibers.
4. Palpate through the more superficial trapezius muscle to locate the belly of the supraspinatus.
5. Ask client to abduct shoulder and resist action.
6. Note contraction of the muscle tissue.

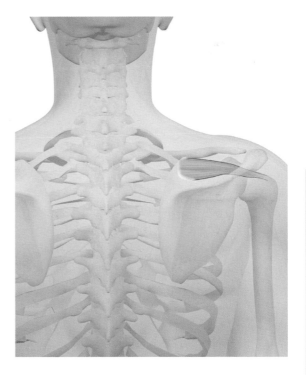

Manual muscle test

Position

Supine. Ensure that the client's arm is internally rotated, shoulder abducted and flexed forward 10°.

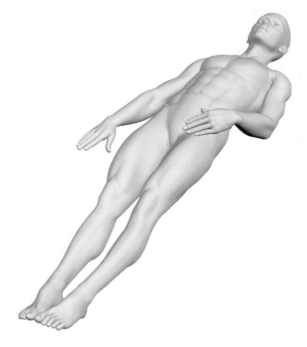

Test

Examiner applies a resistance force diagonally toward adduction and slight extension of the shoulder.

Use an appropriate grading scale to record the findings. Remember to test through the range.

An alternative is to test seated. Examiner stabilizes the superior aspect of the scapula, applies resistance to the distal lateral aspect of the humerus. The client instruction is to keep palm down and raise arm out to the side (laterally).

This will test abduction of the shoulder by encouraging activation of both the supraspinatus and middle deltoid.

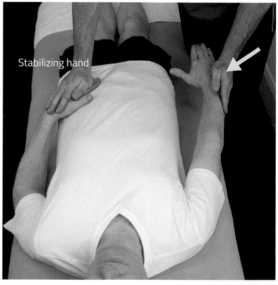

Stabilizing hand

Stabilization

Ask the client to place their hand over the opposite anterior superior iliac spine (ASIS). The examiner then places their hand on top of the client's hand.

Kinesiology muscle test

Position

Supine or seated. Abduct arm approximately 15° with 15° flexion of glenohumeral joint. Client's palm faces their body.

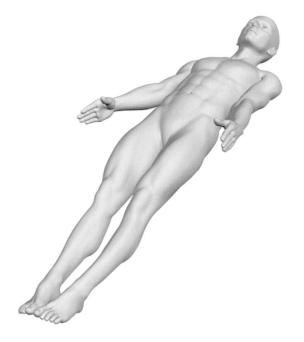

Test

Client is instructed to hold the position of arm whilst examiner rocks their own body slightly, exerting a light force on distal forearm toward adduction, as if to place the arm in the middle of the front of the client's body.

Stabilization

Both arms can be positioned at the same time, and the test performed one arm after the other.

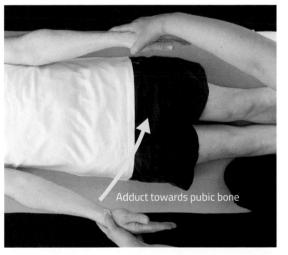

Adduct towards pubic bone

Kinesiological associations

Organ: Brain
Acupuncture meridian: Conception vessel
Emotion: Over-thinking

Video: Supraspinatus

INFRASPINATUS

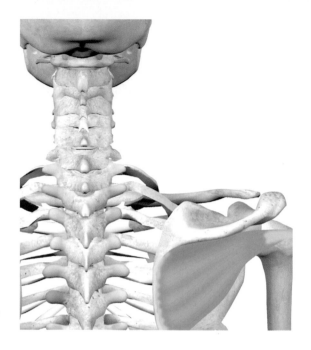

Origin

Infraspinous fossa of scapula and inferior portion of spine of scapula

Insertion

Middle facet of greater tubercle of humerus

Action

Lateral rotation of shoulder (glenohumeral joint)
Adduction of shoulder (glenohumeral joint)
Stabilization of shoulder (glenohumeral joint)
Helps to control medial (internal) rotation of shoulder when eccentrically contracted

Nerve supply

Suprascapular nerve
C5, C6

Arterial supply

Suprascapular artery, scapular circumflex artery

Clinical facts

Works synergistically with teres minor and posterior fibers of deltoid.
Fibers often blend with fibers of teres minor.
Tendon of infraspinatus blends into the shoulder capsule.

Infraspinatus can become weaker or even paralyzed with upper trunk trauma to the brachial plexus.

Palpation

1. Client is prone, standing, or seated.

2. Locate the acromion process and follow it medially and posteriorly. This will enable palpation of spine of the scapula.

3. Palpation is conducted inferiorly to spine of the scapula in line with the directions of the fibers.

4. Palpate through the more superficial trapezius muscle to locate the belly of infraspinatus.

5. Ask client to externally rotate shoulder and mildly resist the action with non-palpating hand.

6. Note contraction of the muscle tissue of infraspinatus.

7. Palpate from origin to insertion.

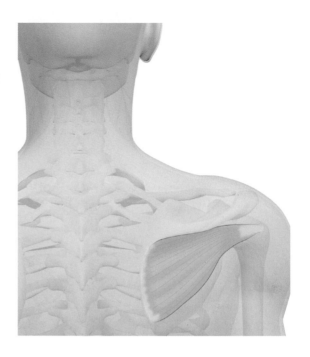

Manual muscle test

Position

Supine. Slightly externally rotate shoulder with elbow flexed to 90°.

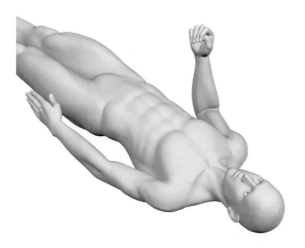
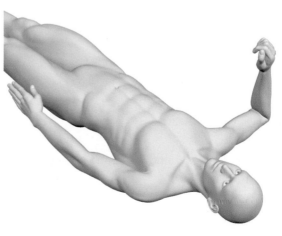

Test

The test can be conducted in two testing positions:
Shoulder at 0°
Shoulder abducted to 90°.
For each of these testing positions the examiner applies a resistance force on the client's arm toward internal rotation.
Use an appropriate grading scale to record the findings. Remember to test through the range.

Stabilization

Stabilization occurs at the elbow whereby the examiner places the non-testing arm over the posterior elbow.

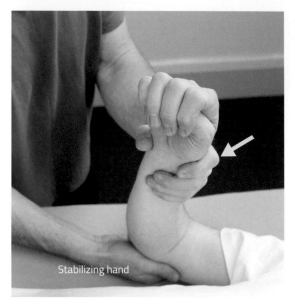

Stabilizing hand

Infraspinatus at 0°

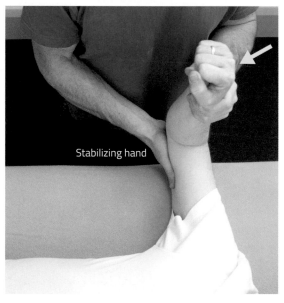

Stabilizing hand

Infraspinatus at 90°

Kinesiology muscle test

Position

Supine. Humerus is abducted to 90° with 90° elbow flexion, causing external rotation of humerus.

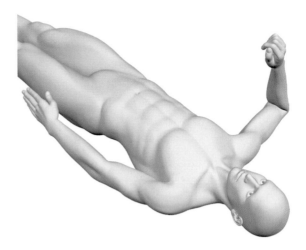

Test

Client is instructed to hold position of humerus, whilst examiner rocks their own body slightly, exerting a light force on the distal forearm toward internal rotation of humerus.

Stabilization

Support the elbow to hold humerus in position.

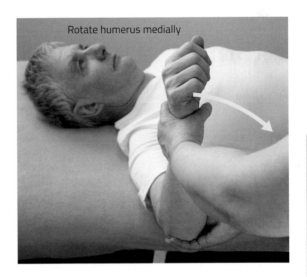

Rotate humerus medially

Kinesiological associations

Organ: Thymus
Acupuncture meridian: Triple warmer (triple heater, san jiao)
Emotion: Stress, anxiety, lack of self esteem

Video: Infraspinatus

TERES MINOR

Origin
Superior lateral border of scapula

Insertion
Inferior facet of great tubercle of humerus

Action
Lateral rotation of shoulder (glenohumeral joint)
Weak adductor of shoulder (glenohumeral joint)
Stabilization of shoulder (glenohumeral joint)

Nerve supply
Axillary nerve
C5, C6

Arterial supply
Scapular circumflex artery and posterior humeral circumflex artery

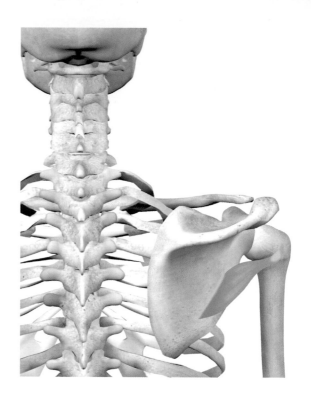

Clinical facts

Works synergistically with infraspinatus and posterior fibers of deltoid.
Teres minor works antagonistically with teres major and its fibers often blend with fibers of infraspinatus forming one muscle. Teres minor is one of the "rotator cuff muscles," whereas teres major is not.

The space formed by teres minor, teres major, triceps, and humerus is known as the quadrangular space. The axillary nerve and circumflex artery run through this space and may become entrapped resulting in a condition known as quadrangular space syndrome.

Palpation

1. Client is prone, standing, or seated.
2. Place palpating fingers along fiber direction between lateral border of scapula and greater tubercle of humerus.
3. Ask client to externally rotate shoulder and mildly resist action with non-palpating hand.
4. Note contraction of the muscle tissue of teres minor.
5. Palpate from origin to insertion.
6. To differentiate teres minor from major, ask client to internally rotate their shoulder. Teres minor will relax whilst teres major contracts.

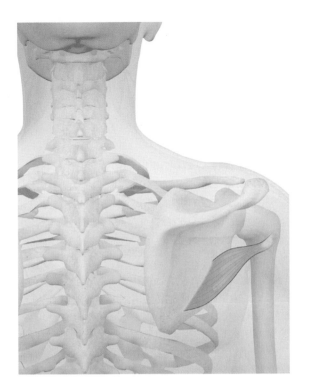

Manual muscle test

Position

The test is the same as that for infraspinatus and can be conducted in two testing positions:

Shoulder at 0°
Shoulder abducted to 90°.
The client is supine with their shoulder slightly externally rotated and with elbow flexed to 90°.

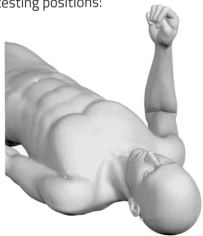

Teres minor at 0°

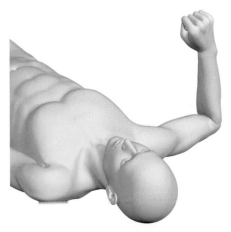

Teres minor at 90°

Test

Examiner applies a resistance force on forearm toward internal rotation of humerus.

Remember: it is important to test external rotation of the subscapularis and pectoralis major before performing internal rotation tests. This aligns with the capsular pattern of the glenohumeral joint. All muscle tests for internal and external rotators should be performed in the two positions mentioned above.

Use an appropriate grading scale to record the findings. Remember to test through the range.
This will test lateral rotation of the shoulder by encouraging activation of both the infraspinatus and teres minor.

Stabilization

Stabilization occurs at the posterior aspect of the elbow.

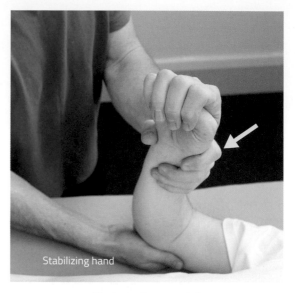

Stabilizing hand

Teres minor at 0°

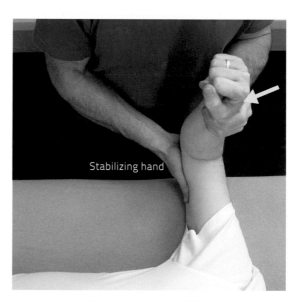

Stabilizing hand

Teres minor at 90°

Kinesiology muscle test

Position

Supine. Flex elbow to 90° and slightly externally rotate and adduct humerus.

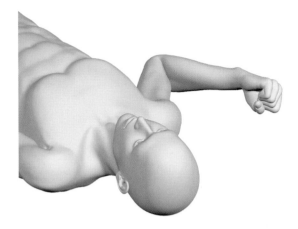

Test

Client is instructed to hold position of arm whilst examiner rocks their own body slightly, exerting a light force on the distal forearm, as if to internally rotate humerus.

Stabilization

Support flexed elbow and hold against the torso in adduction.

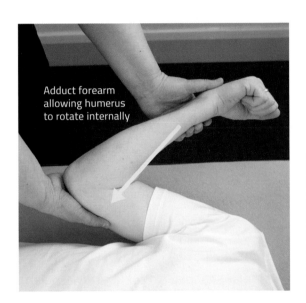

Adduct forearm allowing humerus to rotate internally

Kinesiological associations

Organ: Thyroid
Acupuncture meridian: Triple warmer (triple heater, san jiao)
Emotion: Stress and anxiety

Video: Teres minor

SUBSCAPULARIS

Origin

Subscapular fossa of scapula which is on the anterior scapular surface

Insertion

Lesser tubercle of humerus

Action

Medially rotates the shoulder (glenohumeral joint)
Stabilizes the head of humerus in glenoid cavity
Controls lateral rotation of shoulder (glenohumeral joint) when eccentrically loaded
One of the four rotator cuff muscles

Nerve supply

Upper and lower subscapular nerves
C5, C6

Arterial supply

Circumflex scapular artery, dorsal scapular artery

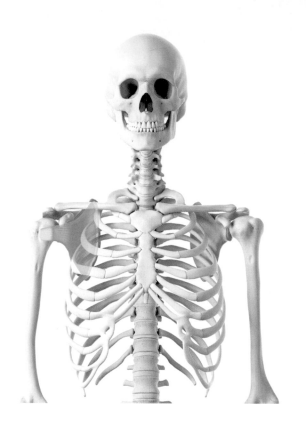

Clinical facts

Works synergistically with teres major, pectoralis major, and latissimus dorsi. Largest of the "SITS" rotator cuff muscles and is the primary medial rotator of the arm. It is deeply sandwiched between the subscapular fossa and serratus anterior. Subscapularis tendon attaches to the capsule of the glenohumeral joint and very little of its belly is accessible by palpation. Subscapularis, teres major, and latissimus dorsi make up the posterior axillary wall.

Upper trunk injuries and traumas could weaken and paralyze the subscapularis due to muscular, vascular, or neurological damage.
Subscapularis tendon is separated from the shoulder joint capsule by a bursa. This bursa is often connected to the synovial membrane. If chronically inflamed, this bursitis could lead to frozen shoulder (adhesive capsulitis).

Palpation

1. Client is seated or supine with shoulder abducted and drawn anteriorly.
2. Rest client's arm on examiner's shoulder.
3. Gently place palpating fingers along posterior axillary fold and direct them inward toward the subscapular fossa.
4. Ask client to internally rotate arm and mildly resist action with non-palpating hand.
5. Note contraction of the muscle tissue.

Note that the medial fibers may be palpated by placing the client in a side lying position with their hand behind lumbar spine and ask the client to relax. The examiner gently curls their fingers under the medial border of the scapula and palpates through the middle trapezius and rhomboids.

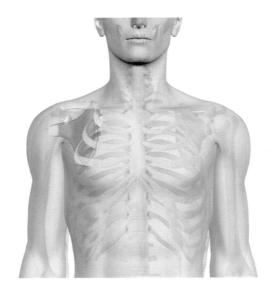

Manual muscle test

Position

Prone. Client's arm is folded back by internally rotating humerus and flexing the elbow so the hand rests on the lower lumbar spine.

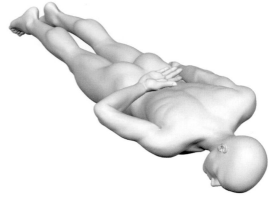

Test

Examiner applies a resistance force from posterior to anterior ensuring the patient lifts the arm being tested away from the body. This is not a test for elbow extension (watch for compensatory movements). Subscapularis may also be tested with pectoralis major by testing the arm in internal rotation with the shoulder at 0° and 90°.

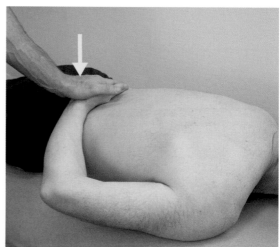

Stabilization

None required.

Kinesiology muscle test

Position

Supine. Shoulder is abducted to 90°, with the elbow flexed to 90°, and with humerus in full internal rotation, so forearm is parallel to the floor.

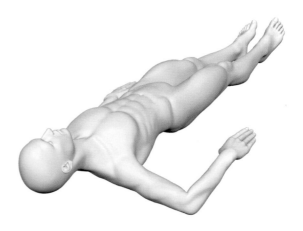

Test

Client is instructed to hold the position of the arm whilst examiner rocks their own body, exerting a light force on the distal forearm as a lever toward external (lateral) rotation of humerus.

An alternative test is performed prone, with shoulder abducted to 90° and elbow flexed to 90°. Examiner takes the humerus into slight medial (internal) rotation and supports the elbow. The testing direction is as if to externally rotate the humerus by using the distal forearm as a lever. Observe for failure of scapula to be stabilized, rather than feeling arm movement.

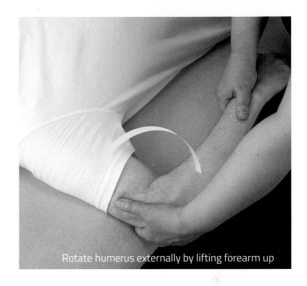
Rotate humerus externally by lifting forearm up

Stabilization

Hold the elbow throughout the test to stabilize. This is a test for ability to internally rotate humerus rather than any flexion/extension/abduction/adduction of the shoulder.

Kinesiological associations

Organ: Heart
Acupuncture meridian: Heart
Emotion: Love, hate, pride

Video: Subscapularis

TERES MAJOR

Origin

Inferior lateral border and angle of scapula

Insertion

Medial lip of intertubercular groove on anterior humerus

Action

Extension of shoulder (glenohumeral joint)
Adduction of shoulder (glenohumeral joint)
Horizontal abduction of shoulder (glenohumeral joint)
Medial or internal rotation of humerus at glenohumeral joint

Nerve supply

Lower scapular nerve and/or thoracodorsal nerve
C5, C6, C7, C8

Arterial supply

Scapular circumflex artery and posterior humeral circumflex artery

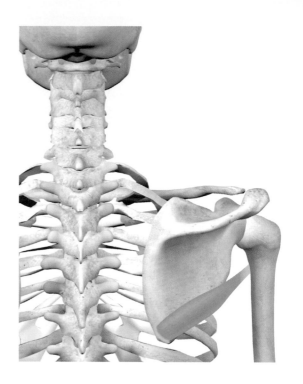

Clinical facts

Teres minor works antagonistically with teres major and its fibers often blend with fibers of infraspinatus forming one muscle. The space formed by teres minor, teres major, triceps, and humerus is known as the quadrangular space. The axillary nerve and circumflex artery run through this space and may become entrapped resulting in a condition known as quadrangular space syndrome.

Teres major is not one of the "rotator cuff muscles."

Teres major is a synergist for the latissimus dorsi and is sometimes remembered as "Lat's little helper." Teres major forms a muscular couple with the rhomboid group.

Palpation

1. Client is prone, standing, or seated.
2. Place palpating fingers along fiber direction between lateral border of scapula and greater tubercle of humerus.
3. Ask client to medially rotate their shoulder and mildly resist action with your non-palpating hand.
4. Note contraction of the muscle tissue of teres major.
5. Palpate from origin to insertion.
6. To differentiate teres minor from major, ask client to internally rotate their shoulder. Teres minor will relax whilst teres major contracts.

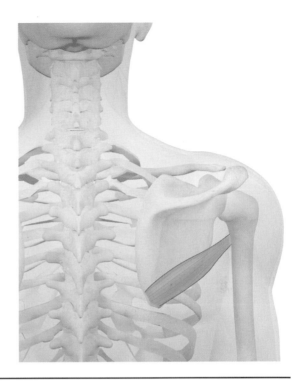

Manual muscle test

Position

Prone with arm externally rotated and flexed with dorsum of hand resting on lumbar spine.

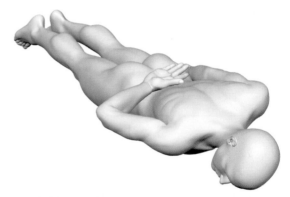

Test

Examiner then applies a resistance force toward abduction of the shoulder.

Stabilization

Stabilization is over the opposite scapula.

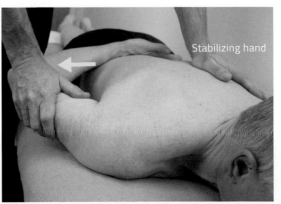

Stabilizing hand

Kinesiology muscle test

Position

Prone. Internally rotate the arms and place both hands on sacrum with flexed elbows, if patient mobility allows. Extend both humerus back, keeping hands on sacrum.

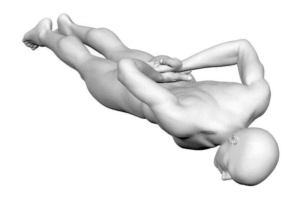

Test

Ask client to hold this position. Practitioner holds the elbows lightly, rocking their own body slightly as if to flex the arms forward. Can be tested bilaterally or unilaterally.

Stabilization

Client stabilizes by placing back of hands on sacrum. Practitioner can stabilize if needed by placing one of their elbows lightly on the client's hands to secure them.

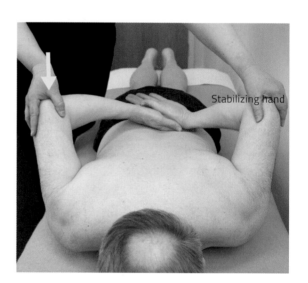

Stabilizing hand

Kinesiological associations

Organ: Spine
Acupuncture meridian: Governing meridian
Emotion: Stress

Video: Teres major

DELTOID (anterior fibers)

The deltoid group comprises one muscle with three different fiber orientations: anterior, middle, and posterior.

Origin

Lateral third of clavicle, acromion, and spine of scapula

Insertion

Deltoid tuberosity of humerus

Action

All fibers
Abduct the shoulder at glenohumeral joint
Controls adduction of the shoulder at glenohumeral joint when eccentrically loaded
Anterior fibers
Flex the shoulder at glenohumeral joint
Medially rotate shoulder at glenohumeral joint
Horizontally adduct the shoulder at glenohumeral joint

Nerve supply

Axillary nerve
C5, C6

Arterial supply

Posterior and anterior humeral circumflex artery
Deltoid branch of thoracoacromial artery

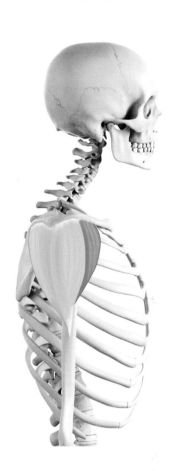

Clinical facts

Works synergistically with supraspinatus for abduction, coracobrachialis, pectoralis major, and biceps brachii for forward flexion of glenohumeral joint.

Anterior deltoid fibers are strong flexors and considered as prime mover for glenohumeral flexion. The anterior and posterior deltoid fibers act to stabilize the middle deltoid fibers during glenohumeral abduction.

Deltoid and supraspinatus are involved in the full range of motion for the shoulder. Deltoids could be weakened through dislocation of the shoulder (glenohumeral joint) and/or fracture to the surgical neck of the humerus which may damage the axillary nerve.

Palpation

1. Client is seated or standing with their hand carefully positioned over lumbar spine.

2. Place palpating fingers over anterior deltoid fibers.

3. Instruct the client to flex the humerus at the glenohumeral joint, thus activating anterior deltoid fibers.

4. Note the contraction within the muscle tissue. Remember to palpate from origin to insertion.

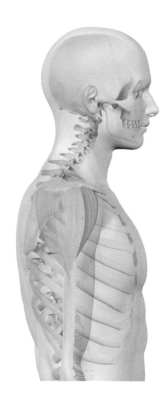

Manual muscle test

Position

Supine with the shoulder abducted to 90°
and elbow flexed to 90°.

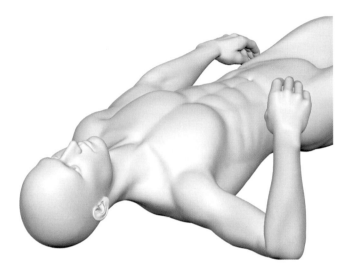

Test

The examiner applies a resistance force
inferiorly toward the floor.

Use an appropriate grading scale to record
the findings. Remember to test through the
range.

A midrange test can be used to assess
isometric strength, wherein the client is
instructed to hold the position without
a resistant force being applied by the
examiner.

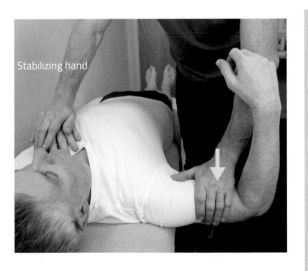

Stabilizing hand

Stabilization

Examiner can stabilize movement by placing
a supporting hand on the contralateral
shoulder.

Deltoid (anterior fibers)

Kinesiology muscle test

Position

Supine or seated.
Glenohumeral joint is forward flexed to approximately 30–45°, with a straight arm.

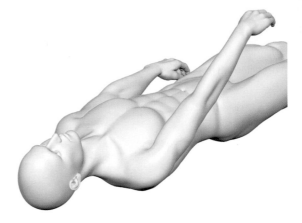

Test

Client is instructed to hold this position, whilst examiner slightly rocks their own body, exerting a light force on distal forearm as if to move the arm toward extension. It is hard to isolate only the anterior deltoid fibers as all its synergists may become involved.

Stabilization

None required.

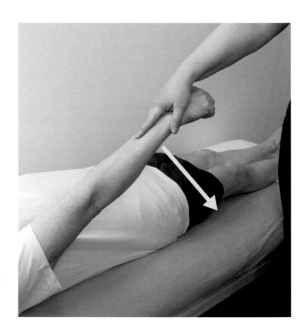

Kinesiological associations

Organ: Gall bladder
Acupuncture meridian: Gall bladder
Emotion: Irritation, stress

Video: Deltoid (anterior fibers)

DELTOID (middle fibers)

The deltoid group comprises one muscle with three different fiber orientations: anterior, middle, and posterior.

Origin
Lateral third of clavicle, acromion, and spine of scapula

Insertion
Deltoid tuberosity of humerus
All fibers
Abduct the shoulder at glenohumeral joint
Controls adduction of the shoulder at glenohumeral joint when eccentrically loaded
Middle fibers
Flex the shoulder at glenohumeral joint
Medially rotate shoulder at glenohumeral joint
Horizontally adduct the shoulder at glenohumeral joint

Nerve supply
Axillary nerve
C5, C6

Arterial supply
Posterior and anterior humeral circumflex artery
Deltoid branch of thoracoacromial artery

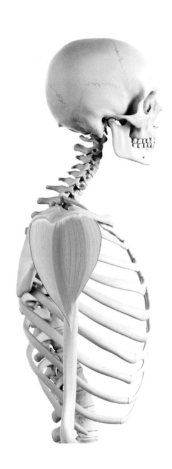

Clinical facts

The middle fibers are strong glenohumeral joint abductors. The anterior and posterior fibers act to stabilize the middle fibers during glenohumeral joint abduction.

The deltoids could be weakened through dislocation of the GHJ, resulting from fracture to the surgical neck of the humerus, which may damage the axillary nerve.

Palpation

1. Client is seated or standing with their hand carefully positioned over the lumbar spine.
2. Place palpating fingers over the middle deltoid fibers.
3. Instruct the client to perform abduction of the glenohumeral joint by moving elbow outward.
4. Note the contraction within the muscle tissue. Remember to palpate from origin to insertion.

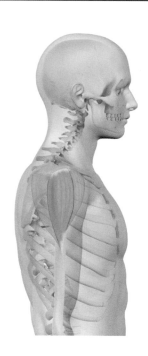

Manual muscle test

Position

Glenohumeral joint/shoulder complex is abducted to 90° with elbow flexed to 90°.

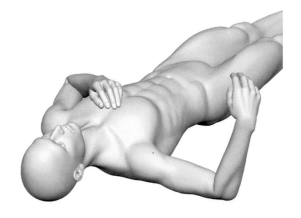

Test

The examiner applies a resistance force on the arm to move it inferiorly into adduction. Use an appropriate grading scale to record the findings. Remember to test through the range.

A midrange test can be used to assess isometric strength, wherein the client is instructed to hold the position without a resistant force being applied by the examiner.

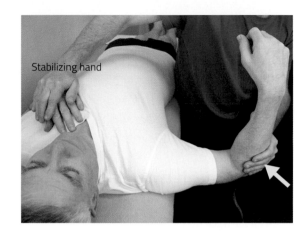

Stabilizing hand

Stabilization

The examiner can stabilize the movement by placing a supporting hand on the contralateral shoulder for the middle deltoid fiber tests.

Kinesiology muscle test

Position

Seated, supine, or prone.
Glenohumeral joint is abducted to 90°, with the elbow bent at 90°. If a longer lever is required or the test is performed prone, keep the arm straight.

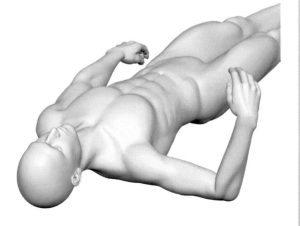

Deltoid (middle fibers)

Test

Client is instructed to hold this position, whilst examiner slightly rocks their own body, exerting a light force on elbow (or distal forearm if prone) as if to adduct the arm. It is hard to isolate only the middle deltoid fibers as all its synergists may become involved.

Stabilization

Support the distal forearm if the elbow is bent.

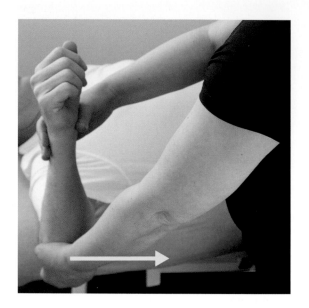

Kinesiological associations

Organ: Lung
Acupuncture meridian: Lung
Emotion: Grief

Video: Deltoid (middle fibers)

DELTOID (posterior fibers)

The deltoid group comprises one muscle with three different fiber orientations: anterior, middle, and posterior.

Origin

Lateral third of clavicle, acromion, and spine of scapula

Insertion

Deltoid tuberosity of humerus
All fibers
Abduct the shoulder at glenohumeral joint
Posterior fibers
Shoulder extension (most active in hyperextension, i.e. extending the arm behind the hips)
Shoulder horizontal abduction (most active when shoulder is in internal rotation)
Shoulder external rotation

Nerve supply

Axillary nerve
C5, C6

Arterial supply

Posterior and anterior humeral circumflex artery
Deltoid branch of thoracoacromial artery

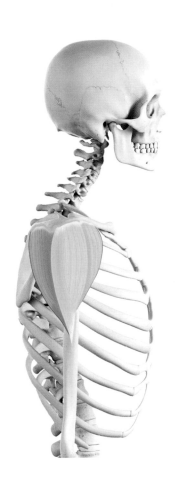

Clinical facts

Contraction of posterior fibers plays an important role in glenohumeral extension. Deltoids could be weakened through dislocation of the glenohumeral joint or fracture to the surgical neck of the humerus, both of which may damage the axillary nerve.

Palpation

1. Client is seated or standing with their hand carefully positioned over the lumbar spine.
2. Place palpating fingers over the fibers in the region being assessed (anterior, middle, or posterior).
3. Instruct the client to bring the glenohumeral joint into extension, bringing the arm backward.
4. Note the contraction within the muscle tissue. Remember to palpate from origin to insertion.

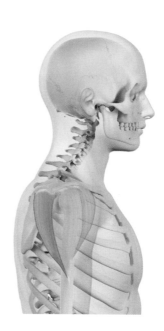

Manual muscle test

Position

Supine.
Glenohumeral joint/shoulder complex is abducted to 90° with elbow flexed to 90°.

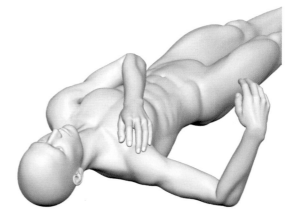

Test

The examiner applies a resistance force on the arm toward the ceiling, encouraging horizontal adduction.

Use an appropriate grading scale to record the findings. Remember to test through the range.

A midrange test can be used to assess isometric strength, wherein the client is instructed to hold the position without a resistant force being applied by the examiner.

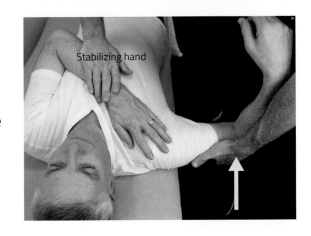

Stabilizing hand

Stabilization

A supportive hand can be placed on the ipsilateral shoulder.

Kinesiology muscle test

Position

Seated or supine. Flex the elbow to 90° and slightly internally (medially) rotate the humerus.

Bring the elbow back into slight hyperextension of the GHJ so the origin and insertion of the posterior deltoid fibers are closer together.

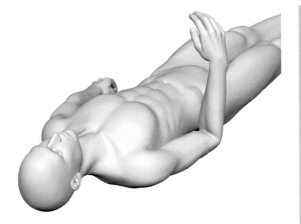

Deltoid posterior fibers)

Test

Client is instructed to hold this position, whilst examiner slightly rocks their own body, exerting a light force on elbow and distal humerus as if to slightly flex and adduct the arm. It is hard to isolate only the posterior deltoid fibers as all its synergists may become involved.

Stabilization

Ipsilateral shoulder or wrist can be supported by the side of the examiner's hand.

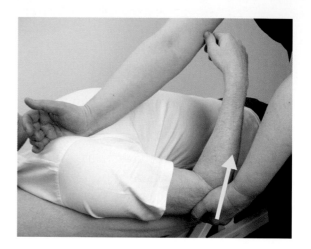

Kinesiological associations

Organ: Lung
Acupuncture meridian: Lung
Emotion: Grief

Video: Deltoid (posterior fibers)

CORACOBRACHIALIS

Origin
Coracoid process of scapula

Insertion
Middle third of medial shaft of humerus

Action
Flexion and adduction of shoulder
(glenohumeral joint), coupled with
horizontal adduction
Helps to control extension and abduction of
shoulder when eccentrically contracted

Nerve supply
Brachial plexus, musculocutaneous nerve
C5, C6, C7

Arterial supply
Muscular branches of brachial artery and
anterior humeral circumflex artery

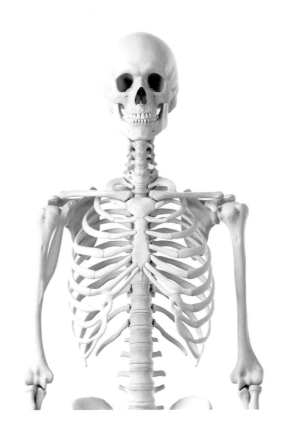

Clinical facts

Works synergistically with pectoralis major,
biceps brachii, and anterior fibers of the
deltoid.
The muscle is a powerful shoulder horizontal
adductor. Despite this function, it is the
smallest anterior arm muscle. It is one of only
three muscles that attach to the coracoid
process. The other two are: short head of the
biceps brachii and pectoralis minor.

The nerve supply to the muscle, the
musculocutaneous nerve, often follows
a path directly through the muscle belly.
Damage to this nerve results in weakness
in forearm supination, elbow flexion,
glenohumeral joint flexion, and numbness
of the lateral forearm. Muscle hypertrophy
usually leads to neural entrapment.

Palpation

1. Client is seated or supine with shoulder (glenohumeral joint) laterally rotated and abducted to roughly 45°.
2. Place palpating fingers over the fibers on the mid medial aspect of the arm and move toward the axilla.
3. Instruct the client to horizontally adduct the GHJ against a resistance force.
4. Note the contraction within the muscle tissue. Remember to palpate from origin to insertion.

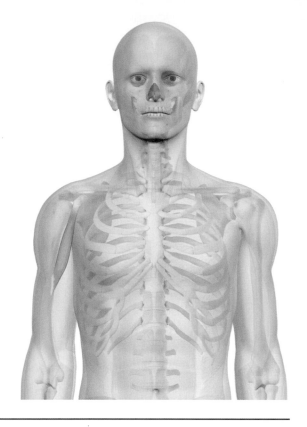

Manual muscle test

Position

Supine. Shoulder complex (glenohumeral joint) is flexed to 45° and abducted to 30° and elbow is flexed to 150°.

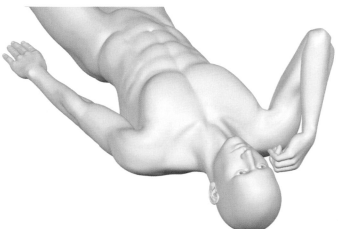

Test

Examiner applies a resistance force diagonally toward extension and slight glenohumeral abduction.

Use an appropriate grading scale to record the findings. Remember to test through the range.

A midrange test can be used to assess isometric strength, wherein the client is instructed to hold the position without a resistant force being applied by the examiner.

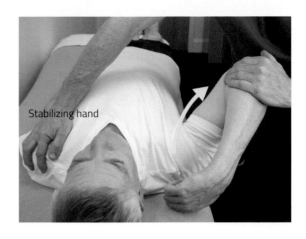

Stabilizing hand

Stabilization

Examiner can stabilize movement by placing a supporting hand on the contralateral shoulder.

Kinesiology muscle test

Position

Seated or supine.

Shoulder complex (glenohumeral joint) is flexed to 45°, abducted to 30° with slight lateral rotation. Elbow is fully flexed to 150° to reduce biceps brachii involvement.

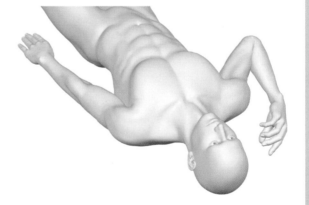

Coracobrachialis

Test

Client is instructed to hold this position. Examiner rocks their own body slightly whilst exerting a slight pressure on distal humerus toward extension and slight glenohumeral abduction.

Stabilization

Both hands are usually used on the humerus when supine. If stabilization is required when seated, the edge of a supporting hand can be used on the ipsilateral shoulder or wrist.

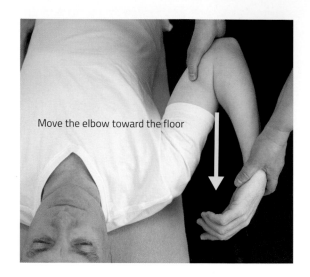

Move the elbow toward the floor

Kinesiological associations

Organ: Lung
Acupuncture meridian: Lung
Emotion: Grief

Video code : Coracobrachialis

BICEPS BRACHII

Origin

Long head
Supraglenoid tubercle of humerus and glenohumeral labrum
Short head
Coracoid process of scapula

Insertion

Tuberosity of radius and bicipital aponeurosis

Action

Flexion of elbow
Supination of forearm
Flexion of shoulder (glenohumeral joint)
Stabilization of the anterior aspect of shoulder (primarily through the long head), whereas the short head is involved with glenohumeral adduction
Helps to control extension of elbow when eccentrically contracted

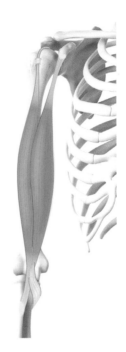

Nerve supply

Brachial plexus – musculocutaneous nerve
C5, C6

Arterial supply

Muscular branches of brachial artery

Clinical facts

Works synergistically with brachialis and brachioradialis to control elbow flexion, supinator for forearm supination, and anterior fibers of the deltoid, pectoralis major, and coracobrachialis for glenohumeral forward flexion.
EMG studies have shown that in 10% of individuals, a third head is visible which arises from the humerus and joins the belly of the biceps. A fourth head has also been seen, albeit this is particularly rare.

In most cases, the long head attaches to the posterior labrum, whereas a small percentage have the attachment on the anterior labrum. Typically, biceps brachii is a powerful supinator of the forearm when the elbow is flexed. This is seen in the gymnasium when working the biceps brachii through dumbbell curls.
The strongest point of the elbow flexion is 80–90° when the biceps brachii is maximally efficient and the forearm supinated.
C5 spinal nerve reflexes relate directly to the deep biceps brachii tendon.

Palpation

1. Client is seated or supine with forearm supinated.
2. Place palpating fingers over the fibers on the anterior aspect of the arm.
3. Instruct the client to flex the elbow against resistance.
4. Note the contraction within the muscle tissue.
5. The muscle can be palpated without a resistance being applied.

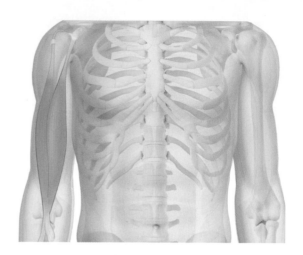

Manual muscle test

Position

Supine. Elbow is flexed to 90° with forearm supinated.

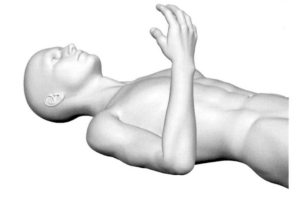

Test

Examiner applies a resistance force in the direction of elbow extension and slight forearm pronation.
Use an appropriate grading scale to record the findings. Remember to test through the range. A midrange test can be used to assess isometric strength, wherein the client is instructed to hold the position without a resistant force being applied by the examiner.

Stabilization

Examiner can stabilize the movement by placing a supporting hand on the client's elbow of the testing arm.

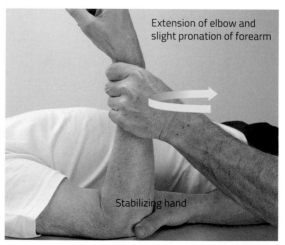

Extension of elbow and slight pronation of forearm

Stabilizing hand

Kinesiology muscle test

Position

Seated or supine. Flex the elbow to approximately 75° with the forearm in supination.

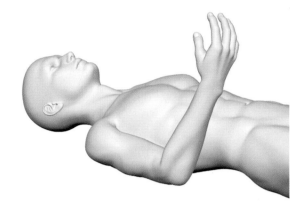

Test

Client is instructed to hold position, whilst examiner rocks their body slightly exerting a slight pressure on the distal forearm as if to extend the elbow.

Stabilization

Support the elbow of the arm being tested.

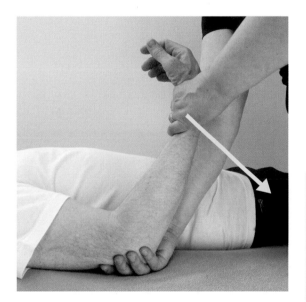

Kinesiological associations

Organ: Stomach
Acupuncture meridian: Stomach
Emotion: Worry

Video: Biceps brachii

TRICEPS BRACHII

A composite of three muscular heads, typically described as long, lateral, and medial.

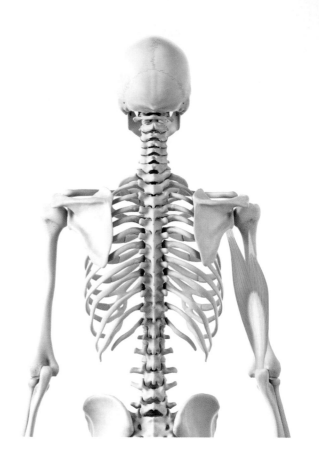

Origin

Long head
Infraglenoid tubercle and neck of scapula
Lateral head
Upper third of posterior humeral shaft above the radial groove
Medial head
Posterior humeral shaft just below the radial groove

Insertion

Olecranon process of ulna

Action

All heads
Extension of elbow
Helps to control elbow flexion when eccentrically contracted
Long head
Extension of shoulder (glenohumeral joint)
Adduction of shoulder (glenohumeral joint)

Nerve supply

Radial nerve. Long head is further innervated by axillary nerve
C6, C7, C8, T1

Arterial supply

Muscular branches of the brachial artery, superior ulnar collateral artery, and profunda brachii artery

Clinical facts

Works synergistically with anconeus. The medial head is the deep head. EMG studies have revealed a tendon that is distinct from, and deep to, the common tendon of the long and lateral heads. Rupture of this deep tendon can cause weakness in elbow extension with the elbow flexed beyond 90°. It is therefore important, when muscle testing the triceps brachii, that the elbow is fully flexed when an injury to the deep head is suspected.

Triceps brachii accounts for roughly 60% of the upper arm mass and is the main elbow extensor. It is maximally efficient when the elbow is between 15° and 30° flexed. The radial nerve traverses the lateral and medial heads and can become compressed or damaged especially when the surgical neck of the humerus is fractured. This could lead to weakness and numbness within the triceps brachii.

C7 spinal nerve tests test the deep tendon of the triceps brachii.

Palpation

1. Client is prone with the shoulder abducted to 90° and the forearm hanging off the treatment couch – forearm should be flexed to 90°.

2. Place palpating fingers over the fibers on the posterior arm proximal to the olecranon process.

3. Instruct the client to extend arm whilst attempting to mildly resist a counter force applied by the examiner.

4. Note the contraction within the muscle tissue and try to palpate all three heads. Remember to palpate from origin to insertion.

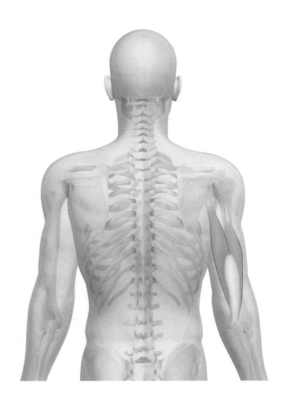

Manual muscle test

Position

Supine. Shoulder complex (glenohumeral joint) is flexed to 90° with slight flexion of elbow.

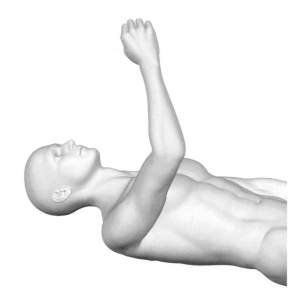

Test

Examiner applies a resistance force toward elbow flexion. Be careful not to flex the shoulder.

Use an appropriate grading scale to record the findings. Remember to test through the range.

A midrange test can be used to assess isometric strength, wherein the client is instructed to hold the position without a resistant force being applied by the examiner.

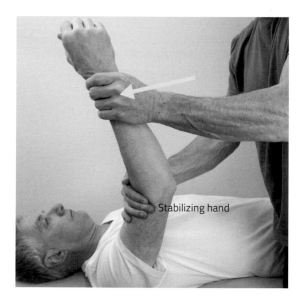

Stabilizing hand

Stabilization

Examiner can stabilize the movement by placing a supporting hand on the client's elbow being tested.

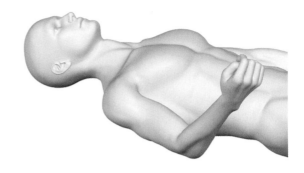

Kinesiology muscle test

Position

Seated or supine. Slightly abduct the shoulder (glenohumeral joint) to 45° and flex the elbow to 30° (15–30° in children).

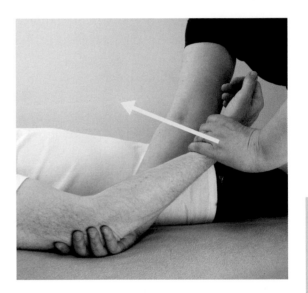

Test

Client is instructed to hold this position. Examiner slightly rocks their own body whilst exerting slight pressure on the distal forearm as if to flex the elbow.

Stabilization

Examiner can support the elbow of the arm being tested to prevent glenohumeral flexion.

Kinesiological associations

Organ: Pancreas and spleen
Acupuncture meridian: Spleen pancreas
Emotion: Worry

Video: Triceps brachii

BRACHIORADIALIS

Origin

Lateral supracondylar ridge of humerus

Insertion

Styloid process of radius

Action

Elbow flexion
Supports the actions of forearm pronation
when supinated, and supination of forearm
when pronated
Assists pronation and supination
of humeroradial joints when these
movements are resisted
Helps to control elbow extension when
eccentrically contracted

Nerve supply

Brachial plexus – radial nerve
C5, C6

Arterial supply

Brachial and radial recurrent arteries

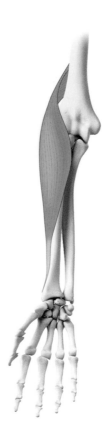

Clinical facts

Works synergistically with brachialis and biceps brachii.
Brachioradialis is the only elbow flexor innervated by the radial nerve.
Deep tendon reflex for brachioradialis tests mainly C6.
Brachioradialis is particularly active during rapid movements of the forearm and is functionally efficient between 100° and 110° of elbow flexion.

The radial pulse can be palpated near the insertion of brachioradialis and the distal tendon of flexor carpi radialis.
Brachioradialis is commonly called the beer drinker's muscle as it is active in bringing a glass toward the mouth.
Brachioradialis was originally thought to be a main supinator of the forearm and thus erroneously called "supinator longus."

Palpation

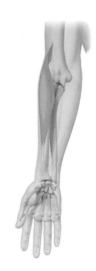

1. Client is seated or standing with elbow flexed to 90° and thumb pointing up.
2. Place palpating fingers over the fibers on the proximal aspect of the radius.
3. Instruct the client to resist a force of elbow extension.
4. Note the contraction within the muscle tissue.
5. Remember to palpate from origin to insertion.

Manual muscle test

Position

Supine. Elbow flexed to 90° with forearm in a neutral position with thumb pointing up.

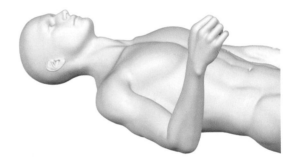

Test

Examiner applies a resistance force in the direction of elbow extension.

Use an appropriate grading scale to record the findings. Remember to test through the range.

A midrange test can be used to assess isometric strength, wherein the client is instructed to hold the position without a resistant force being applied by the examiner.

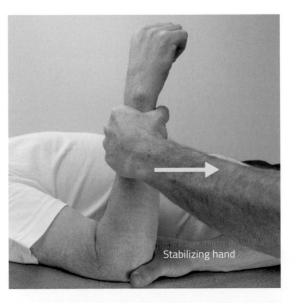

Stabilizing hand

Stabilization

Examiner can stabilize the movement by placing a supporting hand on the client's elbow of the testing arm.

Kinesiology muscle test

Position

Supine or seated. Elbow is flexed to 45–75°. Forearm is in neutral rotation, with thumb pointing upward.

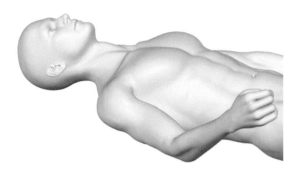

Test

Client is instructed to hold this position. Examiner slightly rocks their own body, exerting slight pressure on distal forearm as if to extend the elbow.

Stabilization

Examiner can support the elbow of the arm being tested to prevent glenohumeral flexion or extension.

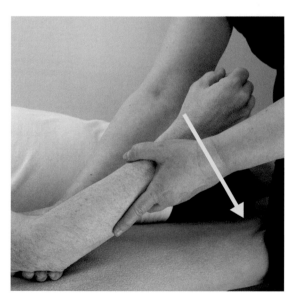

Kinesiological associations

Organ: Stomach
Acupuncture meridian: Stomach
Emotion: Worry

Video: Brachioradialis

SUPINATOR

Origin

Lateral epicondyle of humerus, supinator crest of ulna, radial collateral ligament, annular ligament

Insertion

Anterior, lateral surface of proximal third of radius

Action

Supination of the forearm at the proximal radioulnar joint

Nerve supply

Radial nerve
C6, C7

Arterial supply

Radial recurrent artery

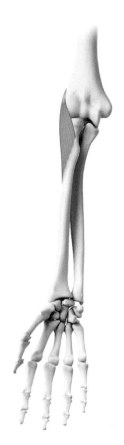

Clinical facts

A small, deep muscle, it works synergistically with the biceps brachii and brachioradialis, and antagonistically with pronator teres.

Fibers of the supinator may merge with the radial collateral and annular ligaments within the articular capsule of elbow.

The supinator has two principal layers, one superficial and one deep. Interestingly the posterior interosseous nerve may become entrapped between the two layers, and may produce sharp, shooting sensations down the forearm when the supinator is compressed.

Used in racquet sports, driving, and household chores.

Palpation

1. Client is usually seated or in the supine position with elbow flexed to 90°.
2. Locate supinator belly by carefully palpating along the fibers and grasping the client's hand in a firm handshake. Execute a handshake with the non-palpating hand.
3. Ask patient to turn palm outward into supination whilst attempting to resist action.
4. Note contraction of muscle fibers and palpate origin to insertion. It may be difficult to isolate the supinator's movement. Brachioradialis contraction is felt superficially whereas supinator contraction is felt much deeper to the extensor muscles.

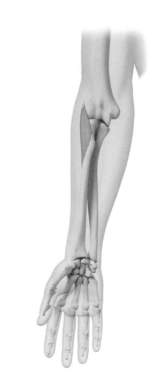

Manual muscle test

Position

Seated or supine, with shoulder flexed to 90° and elbow flexed to 135°. Forearm should be supinated.

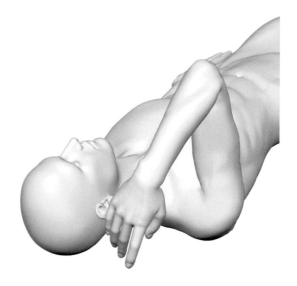

Test

A 75% resistance is applied by the practitioner attempting to force the forearm into pronation – the client is asked to resist this action and maintain supination.

Stabilization

The client's elbow can be stabilized through the test by the practitioner.

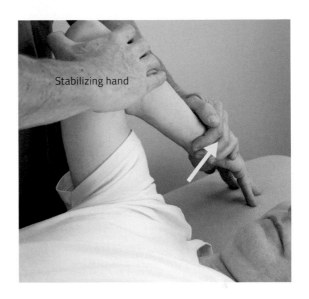

Stabilizing hand

Kinesiology muscle test

Position

Seated or supine. Fully flex the elbow (to remove recruitment of biceps brachii) and flex the shoulder (glenohumeral joint) to 90° with forearm fully supinated. Alternatively, fully extend the elbow and shoulder (glenohumeral joint) back to remove recruitment of triceps brachii.

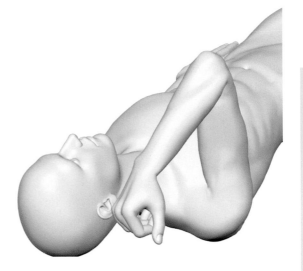

Test

Ask client to hold this position. Practitioner holds the wrist, rocks their own body slightly, exerting a light pressure on the wrist as if to move the forearm into pronation. Take care not to put too much pressure on the wrist as this could invoke pain.

Stabilization

Support the elbow and humerus to prevent humeral rotation when the supinator moves from isometric to eccentric contraction.

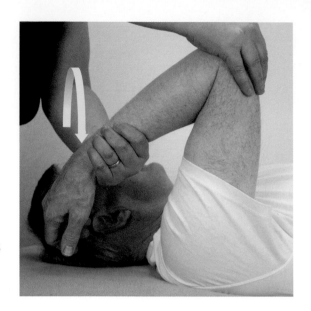

Kinesiological associations

Organ: Stomach
Acupuncture meridian: Stomach
Emotion: Worry

Video: Supinator

PRONATOR TERES

Origin
Common flexor tendon from medial epicondyle of humerus
Coronoid process of ulnar head (deeper origin)

Insertion
Pronator tuberosity at mid shaft of lateral radius

Action
Pronation of forearm at radioulnar joint
Weakly assists with elbow flexion at humeroulnar joint
Helps to control supination of the radioulnar joint when eccentrically contracted

Nerve supply
Median nerve
C6, C7

Arterial supply
Radial and ulnar arteries

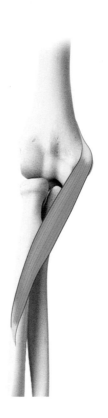

Clinical facts
Works synergistically with biceps brachii and antagonistically with supinator. Important to note the pathway of the median nerve as it traverses the two heads of pronator teres. This could lead to entrapment resulting in pronator teres syndrome and weakness of the anterior forearm musculature, including the muscles of the thenar complex – this is often overlooked by clinicians in considering carpal tunnel syndrome.

Anatomically – the ulnar head of pronator teres may be absent.

Used in swimming front crawl, racquet sports, and daily activities such as turning a door handle and even gestures such as waving.

Palpation

1. Client is positioned in a way to secure slight 15° of elbow flexion and thumb pointing upward.
2. Palpation occurs over pronator teres fibers in the anterior forearm muscular compartment.
3. Client is asked to pronate forearm whilst a mild resistive force is applied by the practitioner. Pronator teres is felt as a solid contracted muscle with obliquely running fibers rather than a soft mass.
4. Be sure to palpate from origin to insertion.

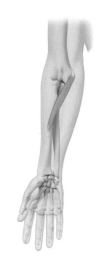

Manual muscle test

Position

Supine with elbow flexed to 55° and forearm fully pronated.

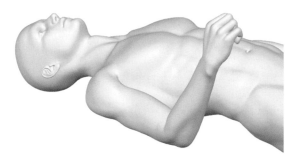

Test

Practitioner attempts to drive the forearm into supination whilst client resists the action.

Stabilization

Client's elbow can be stabilized by practitioner.

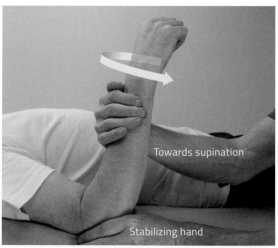

Towards supination

Stabilizing hand

Kinesiology muscle test

Position

Seated or supine, with humerus in adduction, forearm in pronation and elbow flexed to 60°.

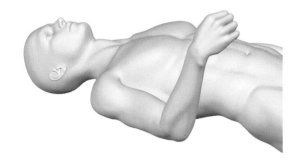

Test

Client is asked to hold this position. Practitioner holds the medial side of the wrist, and rocks their own body slightly, exerting a light pressure on the wrist as if to move it into supination. Take care not to overpower the client or cause any pain in the wrist or forearm.

Stabilization

Support the elbow to hold the humerus in position.

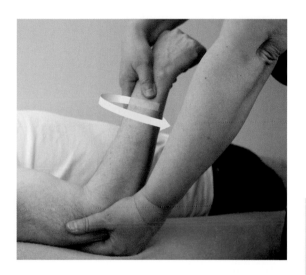

Kinesiological associations

Organ: Stomach
Acupuncture meridian: Stomach
Emotion: Worry, tension

Video: Pronator teres

PRONATOR QUADRATUS

Origin

Medial, anterior aspect of distal ulna

Insertion

Lateral, anterior aspect of distal radius

Action

Pronation of forearm at radioulnar joints

Nerve supply

Median nerve
C7, C8, T1

Arterial supply

Anterior interosseous and radial arteries

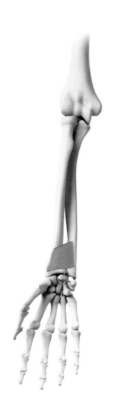

Clinical facts

Works synergistically with pronator teres. Important muscle in maintaining congruity of forearm's interosseous membrane during force transfer in the forearm.
Anatomically, pronator quadratus could be absent in some individuals. Anatomists have reported insertional points for the muscle to include the thenar eminence and carpal bone complex.

Palpation

1. Client is seated or supine.
2. Palpation occurs over pronator quadratus muscle fibers in the anterior distal forearm muscular compartment.
3. Client is asked to pronate forearm whilst a mild resistive force is applied by the practitioner.
4. Be sure to palpate origin to insertion; however, only a small portion of pronator quadratus can be truly palpated just where the radial pulse is also felt. Use slow and secure movements to palpate the anatomical structures, being mindful of neurovascular segments and flexor tendons that encircle the muscle.

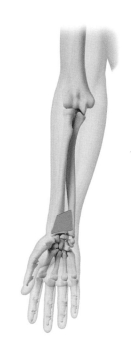

Manual muscle test

Position

Supine, with elbow flexed to 120° and forearm fully pronated.

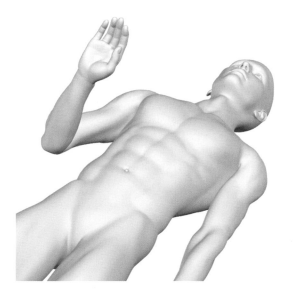

Test

Practitioner attempts to drive forearm into supination whilst client resists the action.

Stabilization

Client's elbow can be stabilized by practitioner during the test.

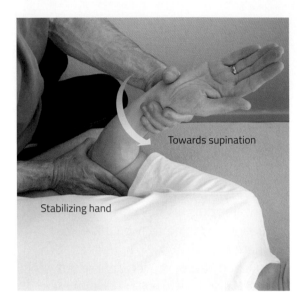

Towards supination

Stabilizing hand

Kinesiology muscle test

Position

Seated or supine. Fully flex the elbow with forearm fully pronated. Elbow flexion removes recruitment of pronator teres.

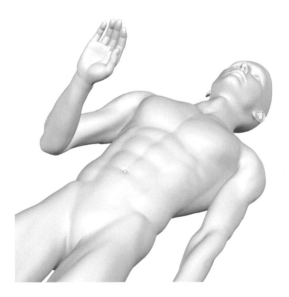

Test

Client is asked to hold this position. Practitioner holds client's wrist and rocks their own body slightly, exerting light rotational pressure on the wrist as if to take the forearm into supination.

Stabilization

Support the client's elbow.

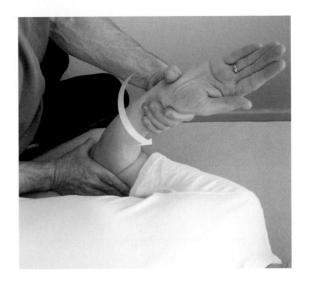

Kinesiological associations

Organ: Thought to be most likely stomach
Acupuncture meridian: Thought to be most likely stomach
Emotion: Not known

Video: Pronator quadratus

OPPONENS POLLICIS

Origin

Trapezium tubercle and flexor retinaculum

Insertion

Anterolateral side of 1st metacarpal (thumb)

Action

Opposition of thumb at carpometacarpal joint (bring the pads of thumb and 5th finger together)

Nerve supply

Brachial plexus – median nerve
C6, C7, C8, T1

Arterial supply

Radial artery

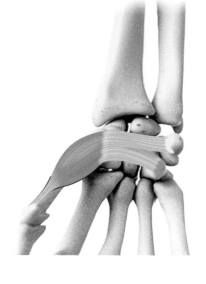

Clinical facts

Works synergistically with thenar eminence muscles of abductor pollicis, and flexor pollicis brevis.
EMG studies have shown that fibers of the thenar eminence muscles can blend together with flexor retinaculum and other wrist ligamentous structures.

Although palpation of the thenar eminence group is relatively easy, individual palpation of each muscle is extremely difficult.
The thumb is in a different plane to the other digits. Opposition of the thumb is really a composite of flexion, medial rotation and some adduction.

Palpation

1. Client is seated with forearm and hand supinated.
2. Place palpating fingers over the fibers on the volar (palm) and lateral aspect of the hand and fleshy padding on the thenar eminence proximal to the thumb.
3. Instruct the client to oppose a resistance force against the thumb.
4. Note the contraction within the muscle tissue.

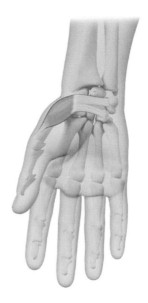

Manual muscle test

Position

Seated. Flex elbow to 90° with forearm and hand supinated. Client brings thumb toward the 5th finger.

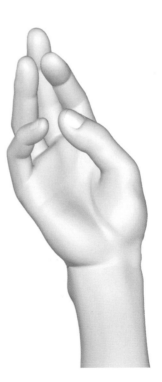

Test

Examiner applies a resistance force in the direction of one or all the actions produced through opposition.

Use an appropriate grading scale to record the findings. Remember to test through the range.

A midrange test can be used to assess isometric strength, wherein the client is instructed to hold the position without a resistant force being applied by the examiner.

Stabilization

Examiner can stabilize by placing a supporting hand on the client's wrist being tested.

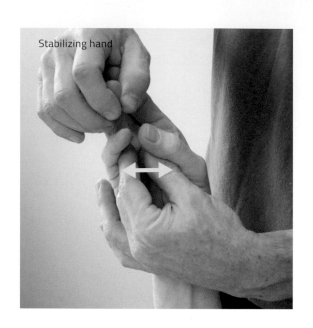

Stabilizing hand

Kinesiology muscle test

Position

Seated or supine. Hand is supinated. Thumb and 5th finger are brought together to form a ring (not a tear-drop).

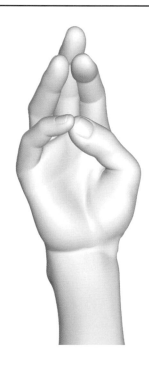

Test

Client is instructed to hold this position. Examiner rocks their own body whilst exerting a slight pull on the thumb and 5th finger as if to pull them apart. Use very light pressure. A small degree of separation is normal. Make sure the muscle attempts to fire and lock. This test indicates possible dysfunctions of the thumb and hand. If performed with hand held in pronation, this tests for possible dysfunctions of the elbow.

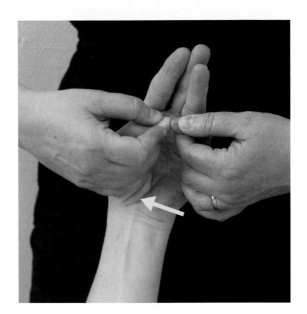

Stabilization

None needed.

Kinesiological associations

Organ: Spleen and stomach
Acupuncture meridian: Spleen pancreas and stomach
Emotion: Worry

Video: Opponens pollicis

OPPONENS DIGITI MINIMI

Origin
Hook of hamate and flexor retinaculum

Insertion
Anterior medial surface of 5th metacarpal

Action
Opposition of the 5th phalanx

Nerve supply
Ulnar nerve
C8, T1

Arterial supply
Ulnar artery

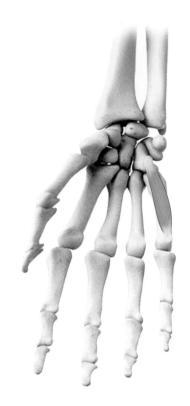

Clinical facts

Works synergistically with the hypothenar muscles, namely: abductor digiti minimi and flexor digiti minimi. Fibers of the hypothenar muscles can blend together to form one muscle mass.
The opponens digiti minimi is the largest of the hypothenar muscles.

Opposition of the 5th finger is a combination of three key movements: flexion, medial rotation, and adduction. Used when grasping objects, writing, using the mouse, picking up small items.

Palpation

1. Instruct client to oppose the digiti minimi against a moderate (40%) resistance.
2. Palpate the lateral aspect of the hypothenar eminence and feel the solid mound of opponens digiti minimi near the 5th metacarpal.

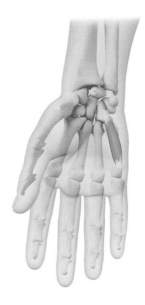

Manual muscle test

Position

Client is seated across a small table with elbow flexed to 90° and forearm fully supinated.

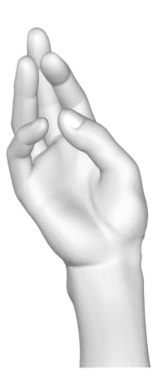

Test

The client is requested to oppose the little finger toward the thumb.

Practitioner intercepts this action by placing fingers in the space between the little finger and thumb. A counter resistance is applied driving the opponens digiti minimi away from the thumb.

The client is asked to maintain opposition against resistance.

Stabilization

Use both hands to test opponens digiti minimi and support forearm on a table or treatment couch.

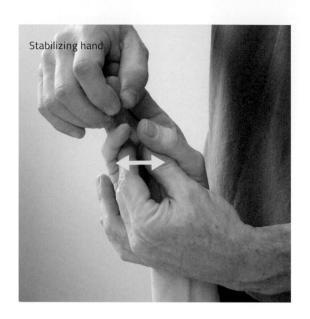

Stabilizing hand

Kinesiology muscle test

Position

Supine or seated. Supinate forearm and rest on a surface such as table or treatment couch. Bring 5th metacarpal into flexion and slight rotation as if to cup the palm. Do not involve the thumb and opponens pollicis.

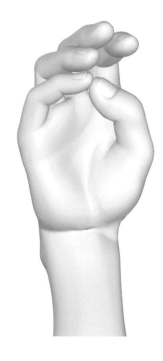

Test

Client is asked to hold this position. Practitioner holds the 5th metacarpal and rocks their body slightly to exert a light pressure on the 5th metacarpal as if to flatten the cupped hand.

Stabilization

Use both hands to test opponens digiti minimi, holding the thumb to make sure opponens pollicis is not recruited, and supporting forearm on a table or treatment couch.

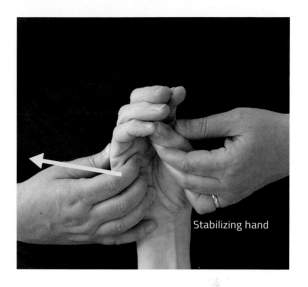

Stabilizing hand

Kinesiological associations

Organ: Not known
Acupuncture meridian: Not known
Emotion: Not known

Video: Opponens digiti minimi

PECTORALIS MAJOR (clavicular and sternal portions)

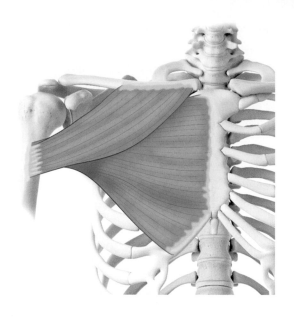

Origin

Upper fibers – medial half of the clavicle
Middle fibers – anterolateral portion of the sternum
Lower fibers – costal cartilage of ribs 1–6

Insertion

Lateral lip of bicipital groove of the humerus (crest of greater tubercle)

Action

All fibers
Adduction and internal rotation of glenohumeral joint
Assists in elevation of thorax during forced inspiration (when the arm is fixed)
Upper fibers (clavicular portion)
Assists in horizontal adduction of glenohumeral joint
Flexion of shoulder at glenohumeral joint
Helps to control extension of shoulder at glenohumeral joint when eccentrically loaded
Middle and lower fibers (sternal and costal portion)
Extension of shoulder at glenohumeral joint
Helps to control flexion of shoulder at glenohumeral joint when eccentrically loaded

Nerve supply

Medial and lateral pectoral nerve
C5–C8, T1

Arterial supply

From thoracoabdominal trunk

Clinical facts

Works synergistically with latissimus dorsi, subscapularis, and teres major for adduction and internal rotation, and with the anterior fibers of the deltoid and coracobrachialis for flexion. The muscle can have multiple attachments on the ribs and sternum, so is an antagonist to itself.

Considered an important respiratory muscle because of its attachments on or along the thoracic wall. The clavicular fibers tend to insert more distally, whereas the costosternal fibers insert proximally. Aids shoulder flexion up to 60°. Pectoralis major is a powerful horizontal adductor and used to stabilize the torso during exercises such as push-ups, bench press, throwing and punching movements. Over-development of the muscles may negatively impact shoulder posture and resulted in a more round-shouldered appearance. Unilateral absence of the muscle indicates a congenital disorder called Poland syndrome which affects males more than females.

Palpation

1. Client is either supine, side lying, or seated, with shoulder (GHJ) forward flexed to 90°.

2. Place palpating fingers over the muscle fibers, carefully feeling the region you wish to examine. Remember to follow the fiber patterns.

3. To fully palpate the contraction of the muscle fibers, ask the client to move their arm across their chest (horizontal adduction) whilst a counter resistance force is applied by the examiner.

4. Note the contraction within the muscle tissue.

5. A more sensitive palpatory technique involves the examiner pinching or firmly gripping the anterior axillary fold whilst the client's arm is in forward flexion.

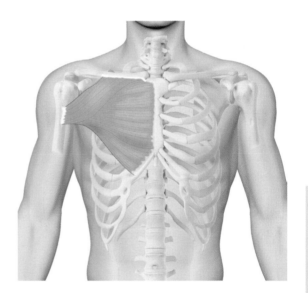

Manual muscle test

Position

For this muscle, the test is delivered in two parts, one for the sternal head, the other for the clavicular one.

Sternal head

Supine, with shoulder (glenohumeral joint) flexed to 90°, with arm fully internally rotated.

Clavicular head

Supine, with shoulder (GHJ) flexed to 90°and with arm internally rotated to roughly 45°.

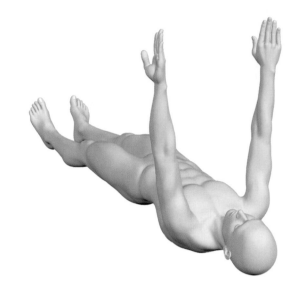

Test

Sternal head

Examiner applies a resistance force diagonally toward abduction and slight flexion.

Clavicular head

Examiner applies a resistance force diagonally toward abduction and slight extension.

For both tests use an appropriate grading scale to record the findings. Remember to test through the range.

A midrange test can be used to assess isometric strength, wherein the client is instructed to hold the position without a resistant force being applied by the examiner.

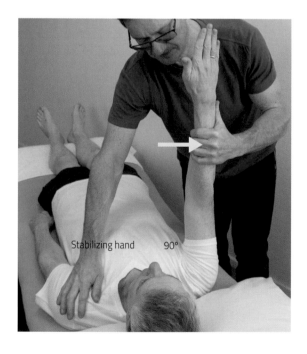

Stabilizing hand   90°

Stabilization

Sternal head
Opposite shoulder is stabilized through the test.
Clavicular head
Opposite shoulder is stabilized through the test.

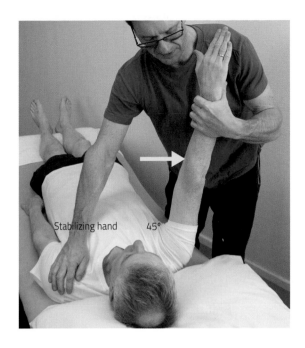

Stabilizing hand   45°

Kinesiology muscle test

Position

Supine. Client's arm is fully extended at the elbow and shoulder is flexed to 90° with full internal rotation so the thumb points toward the feet. Note, there may be anatomical differences in shape of pectoralis major, so always identify the direction of fibers prior to testing.

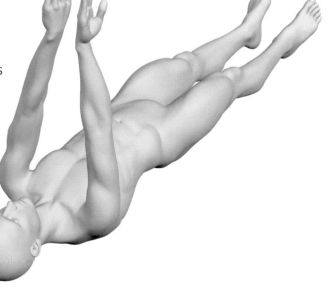

Test

Sternal head (A)

Client is instructed to hold the position of arm whilst examiner rocks their own body slightly, exerting a light force on the distal forearm in the direction of slight abduction and increased shoulder flexion, as if to move arm into a "back crawl" swimming stroke.

Clavicular head (B)

Client is instructed to hold the position of arm whilst examiner rocks their own body slightly, exerting a light force on the distal forearm in the direction of slight abduction and toward slight shoulder extension. Visualize the fibers of the clavicular section and align the movement of the test extending from the muscle.

Stabilization

No stabilization is usually required as the test will be light. Watch for recruitment of other muscles, such as lifting of the opposite shoulder or flexion of the elbow. If stabilization does appear to be required, place the edge of hand on opposite anterior superior iliac spine.

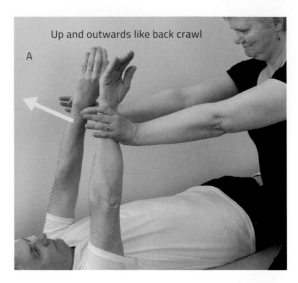

Up and outwards like back crawl

A

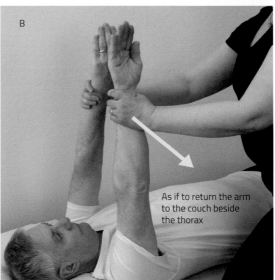

B

As if to return the arm to the couch beside the thorax

Kinesiological associations

Organ: Sternal portion – liver; clavicular portion – stomach
Acupuncture meridian: Sternal portion – liver; clavicular portion – stomach
Emotion: Anger and worry

Video: Pectoralis major – sternal and clavicular portions

PECTORALIS MINOR

Origin

Anterior and lateral angles of 3rd, 4th and 5th ribs

Insertion

Medial aspect of coracoid process of scapula

Action

Important scapula stabilizer for arm movements

Depresses, abducts, and inferiorly rotates scapula

Aids in scapular protraction from a semi-retracted position

Assists in elevation of 3rd, 4th and 5th ribs during forced inhalation

Nerve supply

Medial pectoral nerve, with some fibers from a branch of lateral pectoral nerve

C7, 8, T1

Arterial supply

Thoracoabdominal trunk

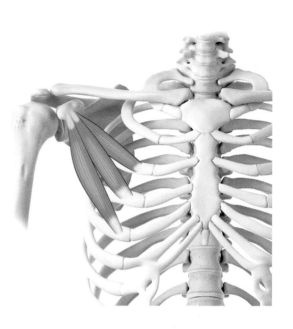

Clinical facts

Works synergistically with serratus anterior. Over-contraction of the muscle may compress part of the brachial plexus branch including the subclavian artery; this could lead to thoracic outlet syndrome.

Like pectoralis major, over-contracture of pectoralis minor could further lead to a rounded shoulder posture.

Pectoralis minor is often thought to assist with respiration because of its attachments along the chest wall. During forced inspiration when the trapezius and levator scapula help stabilize the scapula, the pectoralis minor is then used to elevate the ribs.

Rarely, pectoralis minor may extend to 2nd or 6th ribs.

Palpation

1. Client is either supine, side lying, or seated, with shoulder (GHJ) forward flexed to 90°.

2. Place palpating fingers over the muscle fibers just inferior to the coracoid process. (Always educate the client about why you need to palpate muscles in particular ways. It is good practice to have your client consent, preferably through writing, to more invasive or delicate palpatory methods and techniques.)

3. Ask the client to breathe in.

4. Note the contraction within the muscle tissue.

5. A more sensitive palpatory technique involves the examiner pinching or firmly gripping the anteromedial axillary fold.

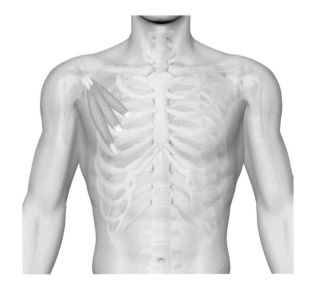

Manual muscle test

Position

Supine. Shoulder is slightly adducted across the body and lifted from the treatment couch. To support the test, client may choose to grip the examiner's upper arm.

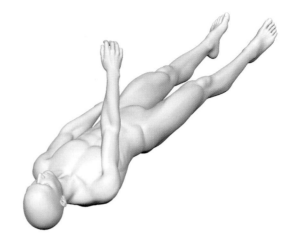

Test

Examiner applies a resistance force toward scapular retraction, using the upper arm to direct the force.

For both tests use an appropriate grading scale to record the findings. Remember to test through the range.

A midrange test can be used to assess isometric strength, wherein the client is instructed to hold the position without a resistant force being applied by the examiner.

Stabilization

Client can be instructed to grip the treatment couch with their opposite hand.

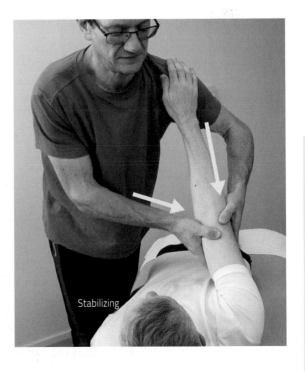

Stabilizing

Kinesiology muscle test

Position

Supine. Examiner passively lifts the client's shoulder off the treatment couch into slight adduction across the body. Best results are obtained by reaching across the client to test the pectoralis minor on the contralateral side.

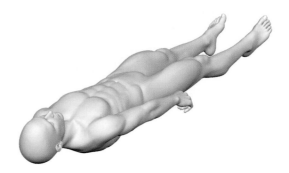

Test

Client is instructed to hold the position of the shoulder whilst examiner rocks their own body slightly, exerting a light force on the anterior surface of shoulder (glenohumeral joint) as if to lengthen the fibers of pectoralis minor.

Both pectoralis minor muscles can be positioned at the same time and tested either individually or together.

Note: look for recruitment of other muscles, such as holding forearm or elbow down on couch, breath-holding, or gripping the hands.

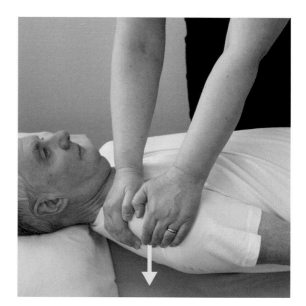

Stabilization

Not usually required as test is light. It may be useful to employ a two-handed approach for the test but maintain a lightness of touch rather than too much force.

Kinesiological associations

Organ: Lymphatic system
Acupuncture meridian: Not known
Emotion: Not known

Video: Pectoralis minor

RECTUS ABDOMINIS

Origin
Pubic crest and pubic symphysis

Insertion
Costal cartilage of ribs 5, 6, and 7, and distal portion of sternum (xiphoid process)

Action
The main action is flexion of the trunk. Rectus abdominis further initiates a posterior pelvic tilt. The rectus abdominis is often referred to as a primary abdominal stabilizer and core strength muscle as it compresses the abdomen and stabilizes the pelvis. It works synergistically with the internal and external oblique muscles Helps to control extension of the trunk when eccentrically loaded

Nerve supply
Intercostal nerves, T5 to T12

Arterial supply
Epigastric arteries

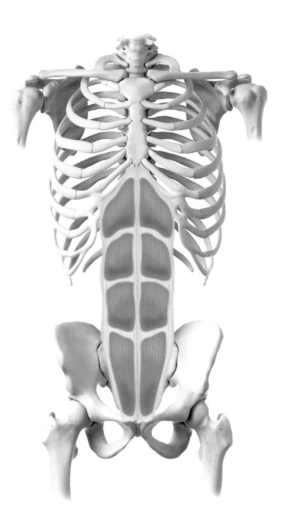

Clinical facts

The muscle is divided into segments by tendinous intersections and fascial slings. The linea alba divides the muscle into a left and right rectus abdominis and is a direct continuation of the rectus sheath.

During pregnancy, the growing uterus stretches the muscles and fascia in the abdomen. This can cause the rectus abdominis to become separated by an abnormal distance — a condition called diastasis recti or diastasis recti abdominis.

Test

Examiner places hand over the client's crossed arms over their chest and instructs client to maintain their position. Examiner rocks their own body slightly, exerting a very light force on the client's crossed arms as if to return the client to the supine position.

Stabilization

Maintain pressure on the feet or ankles with the examiner's knee. Be prepared to catch the client as the testing pressure is applied; if rectus abdominis does not activate on demand, the client may fall backward.

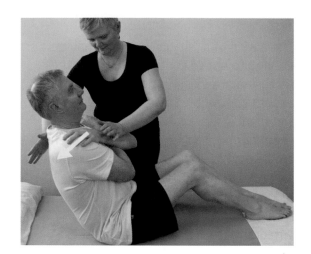

Kinesiological associations

Organ: Small intestine
Acupuncture meridian: Small intestine
Emotion: Worry

Video: Rectus abdominis

TRANSVERSE ABDOMINIS

Origin

Iliac crest, inguinal ligament, thoracolumbar fascia and lower ribs including their costal margins

Insertion

Abdominal aponeurosis (also called the rectus sheath) to linea alba

Action

Together with internal and external abdominal oblique muscles, compression of abdomen and stabilization of the pelvic floor
Raising intra-abdominal pressure
Assists in forced expiration

Nerve supply

Intercostal nerves
Ventral division of iliohypogastric and ilioinguinal nerves
T7–L1

Arterial supply

Subcostal and intercostal arteries

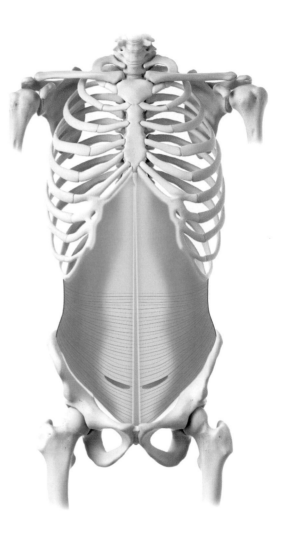

Clinical facts

Works synergistically with the internal and external oblique muscles as well as rectus abdominis.
The upper fibers of transverse abdominis may blend or co-join with the diaphragm.

Transverse abdominis plays an important role in abdominal compression and is activated in daily movements: coughing, sneezing, defecation, and the Valsalva maneuver.

Palpation

1. Client is supine with hips and knees flexed to 90°.
2. Place palpating fingers over the muscle fibers between the iliac crest and lower ribs and costal margins.
3. Ask the client to cough or forcefully exhale. The client can further be instructed to rotate the trunk without flexion.
4. This is a sensitive palpatory test, so it may be difficult to assess muscle contraction.

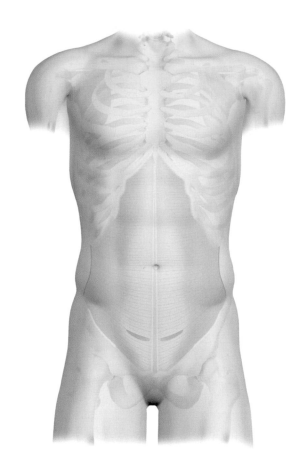

Manual muscle test

Position

Place the client in supine position with knees and hip flexed to 90° with arms across chest. Ask the client to hold this position.

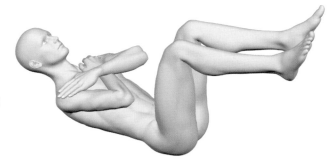

Test

The examiner applies a mild resistance force by attempting to pull the client's knees into rotation.

Use an appropriate grading scale to record the findings. Remember to test through the range.

A midrange test can be used to assess isometric strength, wherein the client is instructed to hold the position without a resistant force being applied by the examiner.

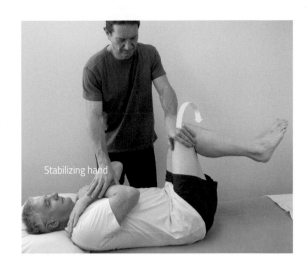

Stabilization

Stabilization occurs over the client's elbows if necessary.

Kinesiology muscle test

Not known

Video: Transverse abdominis

QUADRATUS LUMBORUM

Origin

Inferior costal border of 12th rib and transverse process of 1st, 2nd, 3rd, and 4th lumbar vertebrae
Posterior iliac crest and iliolumbar ligament

Insertion

Posterior iliac crest and iliolumbar ligament

Action

Unilaterally
Elevation of pelvis, lateral flexion of trunk, and depression of 12th rib
Helps to control contralateral trunk flexion when eccentrically loaded
Bilaterally
Assists to extend lumbosacral spine and increases lumbar lordosis
Fixes 12th rib during forced inhalation and exhalation
Helps to control lumbosacral extension when eccentrically loaded bilaterally

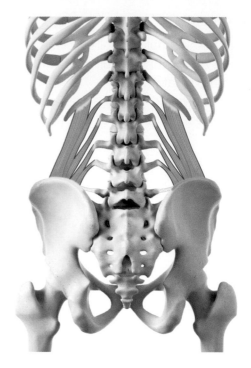

Nerve supply

Lumbar plexus
T12–L3

Arterial supply

Subcostal and lumbar arteries

Clinical facts

Works synergistically with abdominal obliques to affect lateral flexion and with the erector spinae group for lumbar extension. Known as the "hip hiking muscle."
Plays an important role in stabilizing the 12th rib, preventing its elevation during diaphragmatic contraction.

Quadratus lumborum is a core muscle which helps to stabilize the abdomen and lower back.
May attach to the transverse process of L5.
Ultrasound imaging of quadratus lumborum has revealed a second muscle belly is sometimes found in front of the main portion.

Palpation

1. Performed prone.

2. Carefully locate and palpate the iliac crest.

3. Place palpating fingers over the quadratus lumborum muscle fibers whilst palpating through the erector spinae muscle group. To distinguish the erector spinae group from quadratus lumborum muscle, ask the client to lift their head off the treatment couch.

4. Instruct the client to lift their pelvis (hitch up the hip) on the palpating side. Note the contraction within the muscle tissue.

5. Remember quadratus lumborum is a deep back muscle and often difficult to palpate. Take time to locate the fibers.

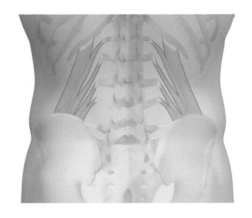

Manual muscle test

Position

Side lying. Upper body flexed laterally and ipsilateral hip slightly raised. The client is instructed to hold this position.

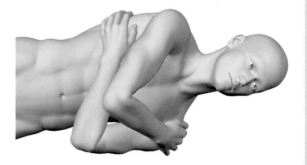

Quadratus lumborum

Test

Examiner applies a resistance force over the client's iliac crest and lower posterolateral ribcage by crossing the hands over. Both hands at this point would further serve to stabilize the mid torso during the test. A further test could involve the patient in a prone position, with the hip hiked up. The examiner then attempts to displace or pull the ipsilateral leg inferiorly.

For both tests use an appropriate grading scale to record the findings. Remember to test through the range.

A midrange test can be used to assess isometric strength, wherein the client is instructed to hold the position without a resistant force being applied by the examiner.

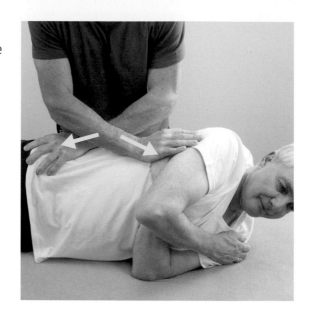

Stabilization

The crossed hand approach used during the test is a stabilizing factor to the iliac crest and lateral rib margin.

Kinesiology muscle test

Position

Supine. Both legs are held together and moved to one side, causing lateral flexion of the lumbar spine. Feet are moved to be approximately in line with the ipsilateral shoulder.

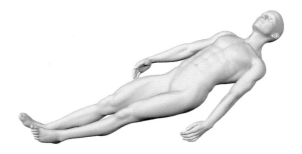

Test

Client is instructed to hold this position. Examiner grasps both ankles and attempts to return both legs to the midline, thus taking the lumbar spine out of flexion. Observe for recruitment of other muscles such as breath-holding or twisting of the upper torso.

Stabilization

Ask client to lightly hold the sides of the couch to prevent swiveling during testing.

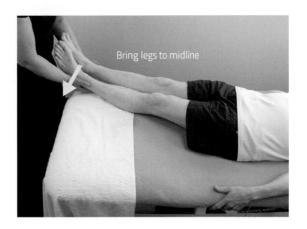

Bring legs to midline

Kinesiological associations

Organ: Large intestine, appendix
Acupuncture meridian: Large intestine
Emotion: Sadness, melancholy

Video: Quadratus lumborum

ERECTOR SPINAE GROUP (sacrospinalis)

This is a composite of three main muscles: iliocostalis, longissimus, and spinalis.

Origin

Via a broad tendinous sheath (thoracolumbar aponeurosis) from the iliac crest, posterior sacrum, 11th and 12th thoracic and all lumbar spinous processes

Insertion

Various attachments at posterior angle of ribs, transverse and spinous processes of thoracic and cervical vertebrae, and mastoid process of the temporal bone

Action

Unilaterally
Assists in laterally flexing the spine to the same side
Bilaterally
Extends the vertebral column and head
Eccentrically, it stabilizes the trunk during flexion

Nerve supply

Spinal nerve (dorsal rami)

Arterial supply

Derived from muscular branches of aorta

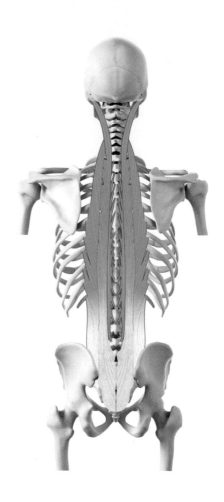

Clinical facts

Works synergistically with some of the fibers of latissimus dorsi and deeper back extensors.

The muscle group is divided into three muscular composites, from lateral borders to medial alignment: iliocostalis, longissimus, and spinalis. Each individual muscle is further divided into a regional segment which further contributes to the name of the muscles, e.g. lumborum to indicate lumbar attachments, thoracic (thorax), cervicis (cervical), and capitis (head).

To remember the muscle order from lateral to medial, it is useful to learn the mnemonic "I Like Standing." This simple mnemonic not only organizes the arrangement of the muscles into iliocostalis, longissimus, and spinalis, but further explains their postural function which is to maintain an upright posture.

The erector spinae muscle group further stabilizes the vertebral column during trunk flexion so unilaterally it can be impacted negatively by scoliosis which causes deformity of the vertebral column.

Erector spinae group is active in the final 30° of shoulder abduction and flexion.

Palpation

1. Prone.

2. It is important to carefully palpate key anatomical landmarks, such as the posterior iliac crest, sacrum, lumbar, thoracic, and cervical spines.

3. Place palpating fingers lateral to vertebral column. Instruct client to hold an extension of the back position. When palpating the erector spinae fibers in the cervical region, it is easier to have the client in a supine position.

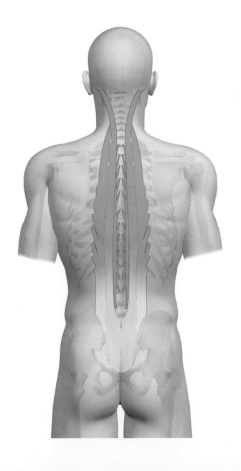

Manual muscle test

Position

Prone with back extended.

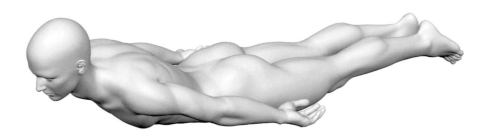

Test

Examiner applies a resistance force encouraging spinal flexion.

Use an appropriate grading scale to record the findings. Remember to test through the range.

A midrange test can be used to assess isometric strength, wherein the client is instructed to hold the position without a resistant force being applied by the examiner.

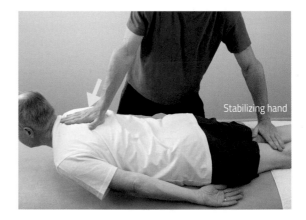

Stabilizing hand

Stabilization

Examiner can stabilize client by placing their stabilizing hand over posterior thighs.

Kinesiology muscle test

Position

Prone. If possible, place client's hands on the sacrum. Ask client to lift head as examiner lifts one shoulder posteriorly away from the treatment couch, encouraging ipsilateral lateral flexion of the spine with some extension.

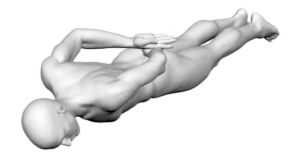

Test

Performed ipsilaterally. Client is instructed to hold the position whilst examiner rocks their own body slightly, exerting a light force on the lifted shoulder, as if to return the shoulder to the couch.

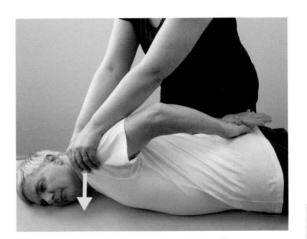

Stabilization

Place one hand or elbow on the client's hands upon the sacrum to secure position. If client cannot extend shoulders sufficiently to place hands on sacrum, allow them to rest their hands on the couch, and stabilize by placing one hand or elbow on the sacrum.

Kinesiological associations

Organ: Bladder
Acupuncture meridian: Urinary bladder
Emotion: Fear

Video: Erector spinae group

LATISSIMUS DORSI

Origin

Inferior angle of scapula, spinous processes of T7 to L5, thoracodorsal fascia, iliac crest, sacrum and 10th, 11th, and 12th ribs

Insertion

Medial lip of humeral bicipital groove (intertubercular groove)

Action

Adduction, internal rotation and extension of shoulder (glenohumeral joint)
Anterior pelvic tilt, elevation of pelvis
Depression and downward rotation of scapula
Helps to control shoulder flexion when eccentrically loaded

Nerve supply

Thoracodorsal nerve
C6, C7, C8

Arterial supply

Thoracodorsal and intercostal arteries

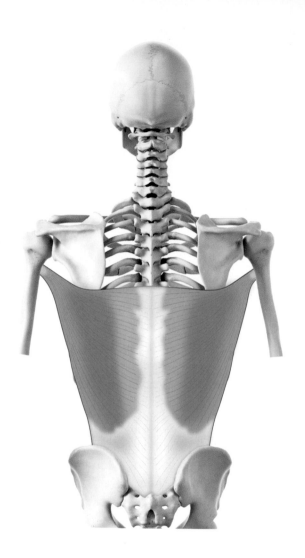

Clinical facts

Works synergistically with teres major and lower fibers of trapezius.

In some people, latissimus dorsi may attach to the inferior angle of the scapula and thus impact scapula action such as depression, retraction, and downward rotation.

Interestingly, latissimus dorsi is sometimes called the "hand-cuff muscle" as its primary action can be likened to the position obtained when someone is being hand-cuffed.

Latissimus dorsi receives its innervation from the upper, middle and lower trunks of the brachial plexus and is only slightly weakened by either upper or lower brachial plexus lesions.

The action of latissimus dorsi enables lifting of body weight and transferring from a stationary to an active position in a controlled manner. This is important for individuals with a disability, i.e. upper body lifting strength is required when transferring from wheelchair or bed.

Palpation

1. Client is seated or prone.
2. Place palpating fingers over the posterior axillary region.
3. Client rests their hand on the examiner's shoulder and is instructed to apply a downward arm force against the examiner's shoulder.
4. Note the contraction within the muscle tissue of latissimus dorsi.

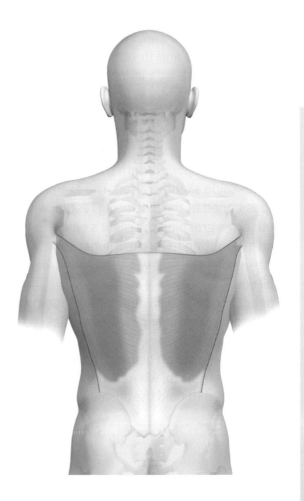

SERRATUS (anterior)

Origin
Lateral aspect of 1st to 9th ribs

Insertion
Costal surface of medial surface of scapula

Action
With origin fixed
Abduction and upward rotation of scapula
(upper fibers may cause downward rotation)
Protraction of scapula
Contributes to scapular stabilization for
upper limb movement patterns
With insertion fixed
May contribute to elevation of thorax during
forced inhalation

Nerve supply
Long thoracic nerve
C5, C6, C7

Arterial supply
Lateral thoracic artery, thoracodorsal
artery, dorsal scapular artery

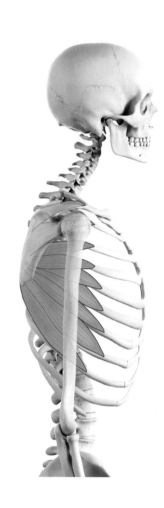

Clinical facts

The attachment of the muscle varies and
may attach through ribs 1–8 or 2–9.
The inferior fibers tend to generate the
most force as evidenced through EMG
studies. These enable an individual to
power through a punch action – hence its
nickname "boxer's muscle."
Clinically, the fibers of serratus
anterior may blend with those of
levator scapulae, intercostals, or external
obliques.
Injury or damage to the muscle may inhibit
shoulder movement as serratus anterior
stabilizes the scapula to the chest wall.
A winged scapula may result from
traumatic damage to the long thoracic
nerve leading to a weakening within
serratus anterior.

Palpation

1. Supine, with shoulder (glenohumeral joint) forward flexed to 90°.
2. Place palpating fingers over the fibers in the axillary region roughly between latissimus dorsi and pectoralis major.
3. Instruct the client to punch forward whilst resisting this movement.
4. Note the contraction within the muscle tissue. The medial fibers can be palpated in the same way as medial subscapularis.

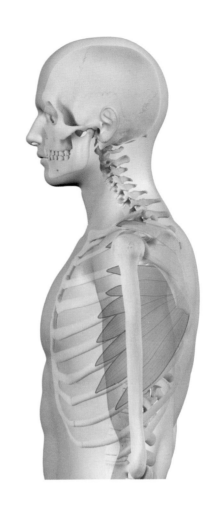

Manual muscle test

Position

Seated with shoulder (glenohumeral joint) abducted to 100–110°, with arm externally rotated.

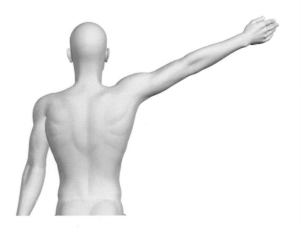

Test

Examiner applies a resistance force on arm (20%) toward downward rotation of scapula (80%). Most of the force is directed through the lateral border of the scapula. Use an appropriate grading scale to record the findings. Remember to test through the range.

A midrange test can be used to assess isometric strength, wherein the client is instructed to hold the position without a resistant force being applied by the examiner.

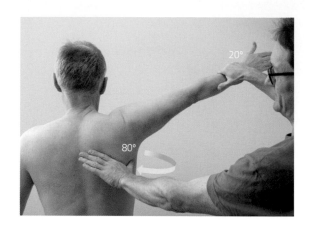

Stabilization

Client can stabilize the test by placing contralateral hand on treatment couch.

Kinesiology muscle test

Position

Supine with shoulder (glenohumeral joint) flexed to 110°. Examiner holds the distal forearm with one hand and places a finger on the inferior angle of scapula.

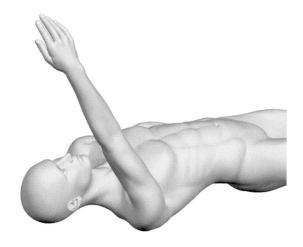

Test

This test is an observation of potential movement of the scapula when the scapula is moved.

Client is instructed to keep the shoulder (glenohumeral joint) still and examiner rocks their own body slightly, exerting a light force on the distal forearm, moving into flexion and extension of shoulder whilst monitoring the position of the inferior angle of scapula. Evaluation of scapula movement is noted, rather than any arm movement. If the scapula appears to "wing" away from the ribcage, the test is deemed to be "weak." If the scapula remains against the ribcage throughout its movement, the test is deemed to be "strong." No movement should occur at the glenohumeral joint. The test can also be performed seated, with the arm positioned in 100–130° flexion with abduction. Position of scapula is noted when the arm is moved further into extension and adduction and the glenoid cavity is moved into superior rotation.

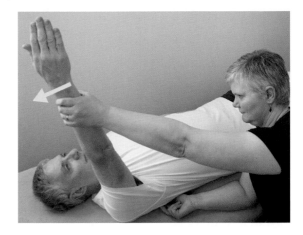

Stabilization

Little stabilization will be required, but if necessary, the client can hold the side of the couch with the contralateral arm.

Kinesiological associations

Organ: Lung
Acupuncture meridian: Lung
Emotion: Grief

Video: Serratus (anterior)

Serratus (anterior)

RHOMBOID GROUP
(major and minor)

Origin

Major: spinous processes T2–T5, and supraspinous ligament
Minor: spinous processes C7 and T1, and supraspinous ligament

Insertion

Major: vertebral scapula border (spine of scapula to the inferior angle)
Minor: vertebral scapula border (medial angle to root of spine)

Action

Scapular adduction, elevation, and downward rotation of scapula
Helps to control scapula abduction during eccentric contraction

Nerve supply

Dorsal scapular nerve
C4, C5

Arterial supply

Deep branch of transverse cervical artery and dorsal scapular artery

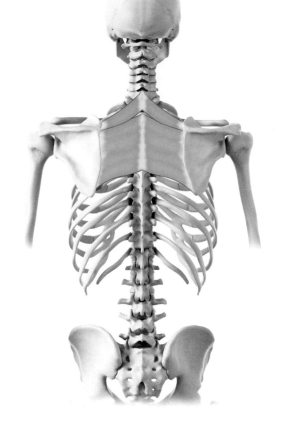

Clinical facts

Works synergistically with middle fibers of trapezius.
Rhomboid major and minor are typically described as two separate muscles; however, EMG scans have shown them to blend together to form one common belly.

This muscle group acts to stabilize the scapula during movement of the upper limb. Poor posture that leads to rounded shoulders could result in over-stretching and eventual weakness of rhomboid major and minor.

Palpation

1. Client is seated or prone with their hand carefully positioned over the lumbar spine.
2. Place palpating fingers over the fibers from the vertebral/medial border of the scapula through to spinous processes of upper thoracic vertebrae.
3. Instruct the client to lift their hand off their back in a posterior direction. If unable to lift their hand, ask the client to raise their elbow.
4. Note the contraction within the muscle tissue.

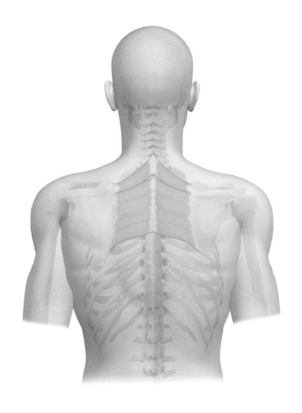

Manual muscle test

Position

Prone with glenohumeral joint abducted to 80–90° with full retraction of scapula. Client is asked to hold this position.

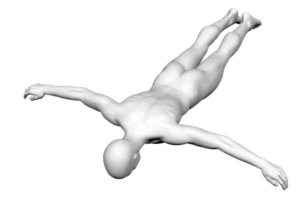

Test

Examiner applies a resistance force over the client's medial scapula by crossing hands and attempting to move the client's scapula into a protracted position.

Use an appropriate grading scale to record the findings. Remember to test through the range.

A midrange test can be used to assess isometric strength, wherein the client is instructed to hold the position without a resistant force being applied by the examiner.

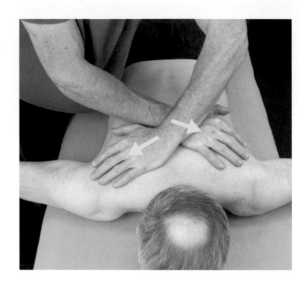

Stabilization

Examiner can stabilize the movement by placing a supporting hand over the opposite scapula.

Kinesiology muscle test

Position

Supine, with elbow flexed to 90° and upper arm held in full adduction.

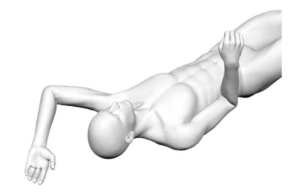

Test

Client is instructed to hold the position of arm whilst examiner rocks their own body slightly, exerting a light force on the distal humerus toward abduction.

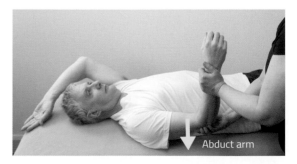

Abduct arm

Stabilization

To prevent cross recruitment from the contralateral rhomboids, place the contralateral arm in full shoulder flexion, so the arm rests on the couch above the client's head.

Kinesiological associations

Organ: Liver
Acupuncture meridian: Liver
Emotion: Anger

Video: Rhomboid group

PSOAS MAJOR AND MINOR

Origin

Transverse processes and vertebral bodies of 1st to 5th lumbar vertebrae and 12th thoracic vertebra, and their associated intervertebral discs

Insertion

Lesser femoral trochanter

Action

Flexion and external (lateral) rotation of hip (femoral or coxal joint)
Flexion and lateral flexion of spinal joints at lumbar vertebrae, bringing trunk toward thigh
Works to produce anterior pelvic tilt through the hip joint
Helps to control extension of hip when contracted eccentrically

Nerve supply

Lumbar plexus
Ventral rami of L1, L2, L3

Arterial supply

Iliolumbar artery

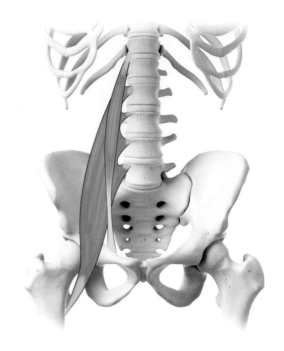

Clinical facts

Works synergistically with iliacus, rectus femoris, pectineus.

Iliacus, together with psoas major, co-join to form the iliopsoas which is the prime mover for hip flexion.

Tightness of the iliopsoas can lead to hyperlordosis of the lumbar spine, known as "sway back."

Bilateral weakness of psoas causes a loss of lumbar curve and rounded shoulders.

Unilateral weakness of psoas causes a lumbar scoliosis. Upper fibers of psoas major may meld with lower fibers of diaphragm at the lumbar vertebrae.

Psoas minor is present in only 40% of population and extends from L1 to superior ramus of pubis.

Palpation

1. Client is supine or side lying.
2. Place palpating fingers gently along fibers medial to the ASIS (anterior superior iliac spine) and AIIS (anterior inferior iliac spine).
3. Instruct the client to flex hip against resistance.
4. Note the contraction within the muscle tissue. Remember to palpate from origin to insertion.
5. Ensure client is relaxed whilst palpating as client's size and flexibility may make palpation difficult.

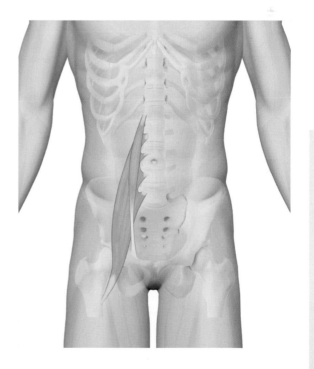

Manual muscle test

Position

Supine. Hip is flexed to 60°, with leg abducted and laterally rotated.

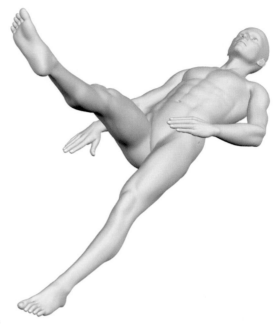

Test

Practitioner applies a resistance force diagonally medial to lateral, trying to encourage hip extension.

Use an appropriate grading scale to record the findings. Remember to test through the range.

A midrange test can be used to assess isometric strength, wherein the client is instructed to hold the position without a resistant force being applied by the examiner.

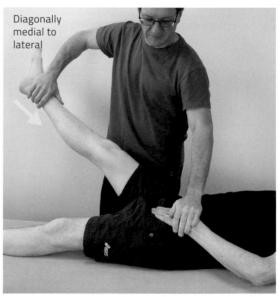

Diagonally medial to lateral

Stabilization

Practitioner can stabilize the movement by placing a supporting hand on the client's opposite ASIS.

It is good practice to ask the client to cover the ASIS with their free hand to avoid any inappropriate or sensitive contact.

Kinesiology muscle test

Position

Supine. Examiner picks up the straight leg from the medial side of foot thus flexing the hip to 60° with leg abducted to shoulder width and laterally rotated.

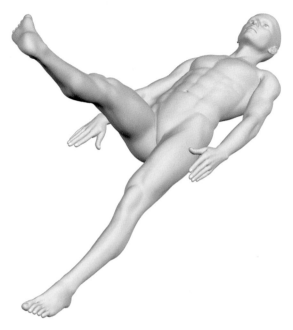

Test

Client is instructed to hold this position, whilst the examiner slightly rocks their body, exerting a light pressure on the foot in the direction of extension and slight abduction.

Stabilization

Examiner can support the opposite ASIS with the side of the hand to prevent trunk rotation.

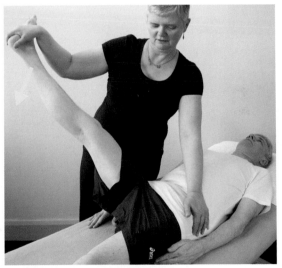

Kinesiological associations

Organ: Kidney
Acupuncture meridian: Kidney
Emotion: Fear/fright

Video: Psoas major

ILIACUS

Origin

Anterior surface of ilium at iliac fossa and sacral ala

Insertion

Lesser trochanter of femur

Action

Flexion and external (lateral) rotation of hip at coxal joint
Works to produce anterior pelvic tilt through the hip (coxal) joint
Helps to control hip extension when contracted eccentrically

Nerve supply

Femoral nerve
L2, L3

Arterial supply

Internal iliac artery

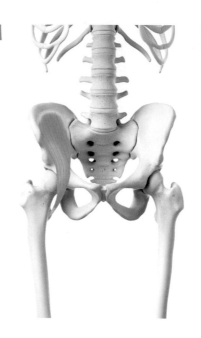

Clinical facts

Works synergistically with psoas major, rectus femoris, and pectineus.

Iliacus together with psoas major co-join to form the iliopsoas which is the prime mover for hip flexion.

Tightness of the iliopsoas can lead to hyperlordosis of the lumbar spine, known as "sway back."

During sit-ups the iliopsoas is often erroneously activated. To avoid this the thigh and knee should be flexed sufficiently so that the abdominal muscles fire and not iliopsoas.

Palpation

1. Client is supine or side lying.

2. Place palpating fingers gently along fibers medial to ASIS (anterior superior iliac spine) and along anterior aspect of the iliac crest and fossa.

3. Instruct the client to flex hip against resistance.

4. Note the contraction within the muscle tissue. Remember to palpate from origin to insertion.

5. Ensure client is relaxed whilst palpating as client's size and flexibility may make palpation difficult.

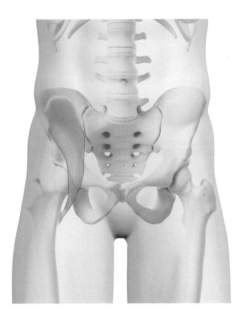

Manual muscle test

Position

Supine. Hip is flexed to 40° with leg externally (laterally) rotated.

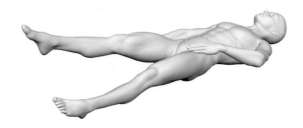

Test

Examiner applies a resistance force as if to encourage hip extension.

Use an appropriate grading scale to record the findings. Remember to test through the range.

A midrange test can be used to assess isometric strength, wherein the client is instructed to hold the position without a resistant force being applied by the examiner.

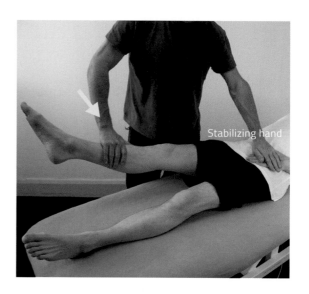

Stabilizing hand

Stabilization

Examiner can stabilize the movement by placing a supporting hand on the client's opposite ASIS. It is good practice to ask the client to cover the ASIS with their free hand, to avoid any inappropriate or sensitive contact.

Kinesiology muscle test

Position

Supine. Hip is flexed to 40° with leg externally (laterally) rotated.

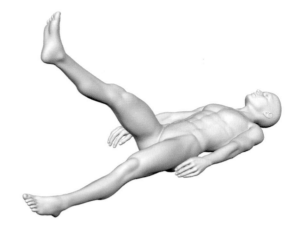

Test

Client is instructed to hold this position. Examiner rocks their own body slightly to exert a light pressure on the foot or ankle as if to extend the hip and return the leg to the couch.

Stabilization

Pelvis can be stabilized by supporting the contralateral ASIS with the examiner's other hand.

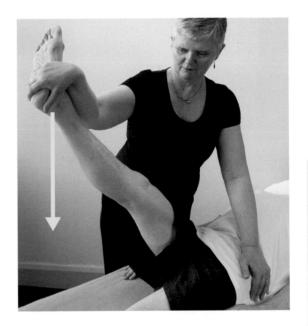

Kinesiological associations

Organ: Kidney, ileocecal valve
Acupuncture meridian: Kidney
Emotion: Fear, fright

Video: Iliacus

PIRIFORMIS

Origin

Anterior surface of sacrum

Insertion

Greater trochanter of femur

Action

Aids hip abduction when thigh is flexed
Works as part of a group to externally
(laterally) rotate the hip

Nerve supply

Lumbosacral plexus
L5, S1, S2

Arterial supply

Superior and inferior gluteal arteries

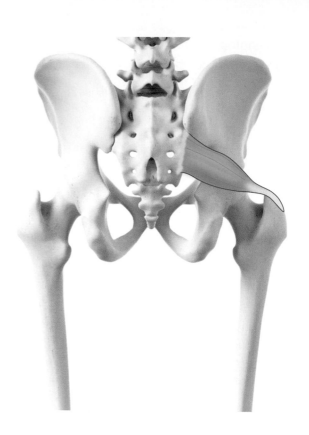

Clinical facts

Works synergistically with lateral hip rotators: gemellus superior and inferior, obturator internus and externus, quadratus femoris.

Distal fibers of piriformis may blend with gluteus medius.

Piriformis is an important site for the path of the sciatic nerve fibers. In approximately 83% of individuals the nerve passes below the muscle, whilst in the remaining 17% the nerve passes through the belly of the muscle. "Piriformis syndrome" is a condition which arises from the compression of the sciatic nerve fibers as they pass through or below the muscle, resulting in sciatic-type symptoms of leg and buttock pain. A true piriformis syndrome is relatively rare.

Palpation

1. Client is prone or side lying.

2. Place palpating fingers gently along fibers between the posterior superior iliac spine (PSIS) and greater trochanter of femur.

3. Instruct the client to rotate hip externally.

4. Note the contraction within the muscle tissue. Piriformis is a deep muscle lying below gluteus maximus. Remember to palpate from origin to insertion.

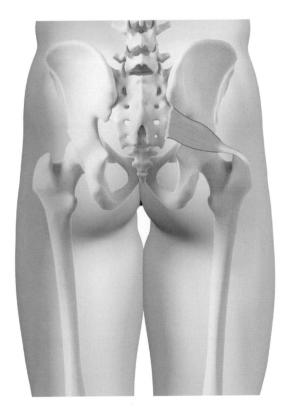

Manual muscle test

Position

Prone. Knee is flexed to 90° with femur externally rotated.

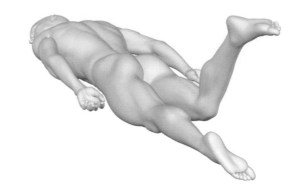

Test

Examiner applies a resistant force to encourage femoral internal rotation by pulling the ankle laterally.

Use an appropriate grading scale to record the findings. Remember to test through the range.

A midrange test can be used to assess isometric strength, wherein the client is instructed to hold the position without a resistant force being applied by the examiner.

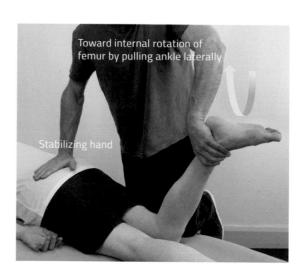

Toward internal rotation of femur by pulling ankle laterally

Stabilizing hand

Stabilization

Examiner can stabilize the movement by placing a supporting hand on the client's knee or posterior superior iliac spine (PSIS).

Kinesiology muscle test

Position

Prone. Knee is flexed to 90° with femur externally rotated, so the foot is moved just across the midline of the body.

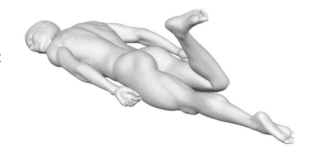

Test

Client is asked to hold his position. Examiner rocks his own body slightly, exerting light pressure on the medial surface of the ankle, as if to move the foot laterally away from the midline.

Client may feel very disorientated in this position and not know which direction to hold the leg in position, so give some proprioceptive input to the medial side of the lower leg and ankle so they are aware of the direction of the test.

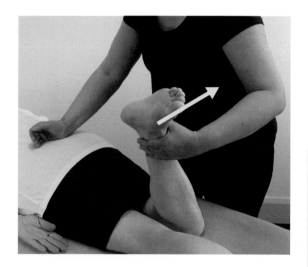

Stabilization

Use the side of the hand on the sacrum to stabilize pelvis.

Kinesiological associations

Organ: Reproductive organs
Acupuncture meridian: Circulation/sex (pericardium)
Emotion: Low mood

Video: Piriformis

GLUTEUS MAXIMUS

Origin
Posterior iliac crest, sacrum, coccyx, and sacrotuberous ligament

Insertion
Iliotibial band (ITB) and gluteal tuberosity of femur

Action
Extension and lateral rotation of hip
Abduction of hip mainly through upper third of gluteus maximus fibers, and adduction of hip through lower two thirds of gluteus maximus fibers
Gluteus maximus further encourages a posterior pelvic tilt
Helps control flexion of hip when eccentrically contracted, such as when sitting from a standing position. An "anti-gravity" muscle

Nerve supply
Inferior gluteal nerve
L5, S1, S2

Arterial supply
Inferior and superior gluteal arteries

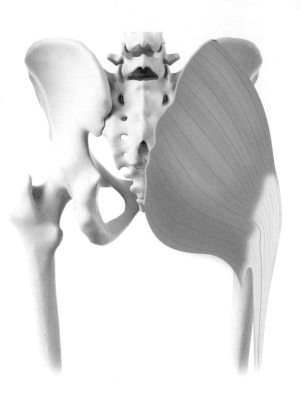

Clinical facts

Works synergistically with gluteus minimus and medius as well as the hamstring group. This is the largest muscle in the body by weight.

The upper three quarters of gluteus maximus inserts in the iliotibial band, with the lower quarter inserting into the gluteal tuberosity.

When standing, gluteus maximus covers the ischial tuberosity; however, when sitting it slides out of the way to expose the ischial tuberosity.

Bilateral contraction of gluteus maximus may contribute to the contraction of the external anal sphincter.

It is important in elevating the arches of the foot when standing predominantly through bilateral contraction resulting in external rotation of the femurs, tibias, and tarsals.

Palpation

1. Client is prone.
2. Place palpating fingers gently along fibers between the lateral aspect of the sacrum and gluteal tuberosity.
3. Instruct the client to extend the hip by lifting leg up from couch.
4. Note the contraction within the muscle tissue. Remember to palpate from origin to insertion.

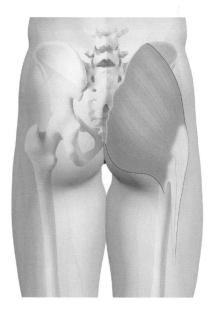

Manual muscle test

Position

Prone. Knee is flexed to 90° with hip fully extended.

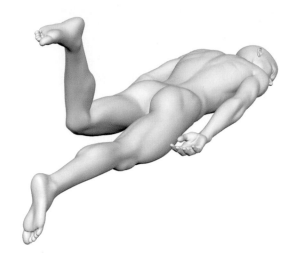

Test

Examiner applies a resistance force to encourage hip flexion – downward into the treatment couch.

Use an appropriate grading scale to record the findings. Remember to test through the range.

A midrange test can be used to assess isometric strength, wherein the client is instructed to hold the position without a resistant force being applied by the examiner.

Stabilization

Examiner can stabilize the movement by placing a supporting hand on the client's opposite PSIS.

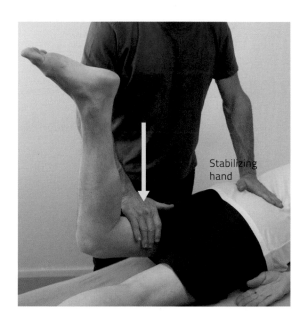

Stabilizing hand

Kinesiology muscle test

Position

Prone. Knee is flexed to 90° with hip fully extended so femur is lifted off the treatment couch by the examiner by grasping the distal part of lower leg.

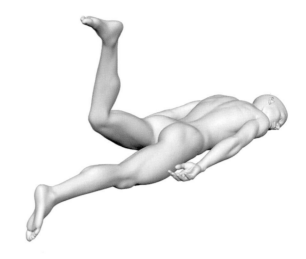

Test

Client is asked to hold this position. Examiner holds the lower leg up with one hand and presses down on the femur by rocking their body slightly. If gluteus maximus is very weak, the leg will not be able to be held in position and will drop to the couch before test takes place.

Stabilization

Stabilization occurs by holding the leg off the couch with one hand and testing with the other.

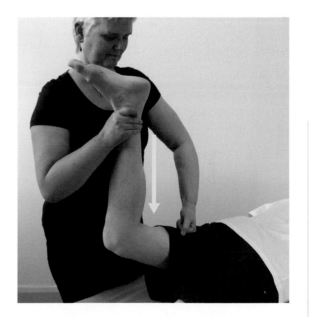

Kinesiological associations

Organ: Reproductive organs
Acupuncture meridian: Circulation/sex (pericardium)
Emotion: Low mood

Video: Gluteus maximus

GLUTEUS MEDIUS

Origin

Outer aspect of ilium between anterior and posterior gluteal lines

Insertion

Greater trochanter of femur (superior and lateral surfaces)

Action

Main action is hip abduction
Gluteus medius anterior fibers work to produce medial rotation and flexion of the hip
Posterior fibers aid lateral rotation and hip extension
Gluteus medius is important in the gait cycle and works to stabilize the pelvis and prevent the free leg from sagging
Helps to control hip adduction and internal rotation when eccentrically contracted

Nerve supply

Superior gluteal nerve
L4, L5, S1

Arterial supply

Superior gluteal artery

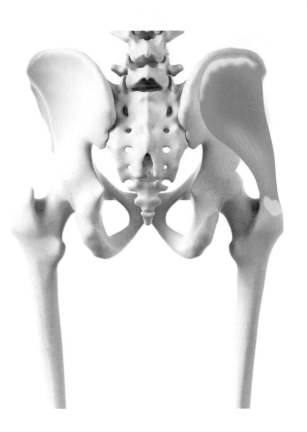

Clinical facts

Works synergistically with gluteus minimus and maximus, and tensor fasciae latae (TFL). The fan-shaped muscle fiber pattern of gluteus medius has resulted in some clinicians organizing the muscle into anterior, middle, and posterior regions. It is encased in the gluteal aponeurosis. The Trendelenburg test is used to assess the function and strength of gluteus medius. If it is weak or injured on the standing leg, there would be a marked sagging on the opposite side and the client may walk with a distinctive dropped hip, called "Trendelenburg gait."

Gluteus medius is often thought to be the "deltoid of the hip" due to its multiple actions.

Tightness of gluteus medius could result in a functionally shorter leg described by clinicians as a compensatory scoliosis.

Palpation

1. Client is prone or side lying.
2. Place palpating fingers gently along gluteus medius fibers between the iliac crest and greater trochanter.
3. Instruct the client to abduct the hip.
4. Note the contraction within the muscle tissue. Remember to palpate from origin to insertion.
5. It is often difficult to distinguish the gluteus medius fibers from the TFL and posterior fibers of gluteus maximus.

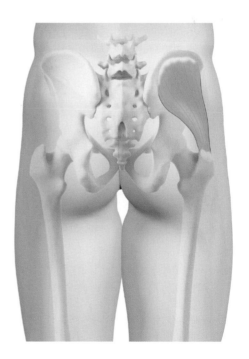

Manual muscle test

Position

Supine. Hip is flexed to 5° with slight abduction.

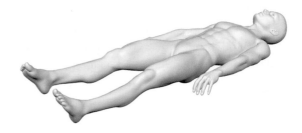

Test

Examiner applies a resistance force diagonally toward opposite ankle to encourage hip adduction.
Use an appropriate grading scale to record the findings. Remember to test through the range.
A midrange test can be used to assess isometric strength, wherein the client is instructed to hold the position without a resistant force being applied by the examiner.

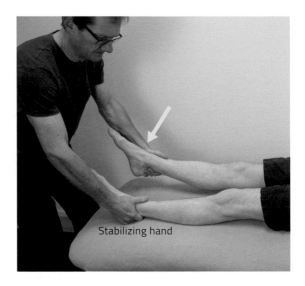

Stabilizing hand

Stabilization

Examiner can stabilize the movement by placing a supporting hand on client's opposite ankle.

Kinesiology muscle test

Position

Supine. Client abducts leg to shoulder width, with examiner lifting the leg slightly so the calf clears the couch. Medially rotate the leg.

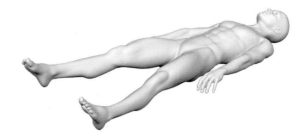

Test

Client is asked to hold this position. Examiner rocks their body slightly, exerting light pressure on the lateral side of ankle as if to adduct the leg in medial rotation.

Stabilization

Examiner can hold the opposite ankle.

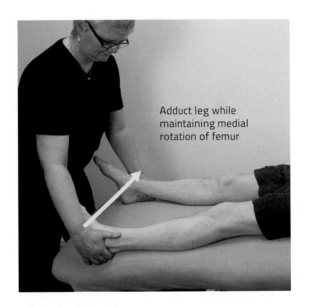

Adduct leg while maintaining medial rotation of femur

Kinesiological associations

Organ: Reproductive organs
Acupuncture meridian: Circulation/sex (pericardium)
Emotion: Low mood

Video: Gluteus medius

TENSOR FASCIAE LATAE

Origin

Iliac crest, posterior (PSIS) to anterior superior iliac spine (ASIS)

Insertion

Iliotibial band (ITB) – distal to greater trochanter

Action

Flexion, abduction and internal rotation of the hip (anterior pelvic tilt)
Serves to tense the ITB to support the femur whilst standing
Helps to control lateral rotation and extension of the hip when eccentrically contracted

Nerve supply

Superior gluteal nerve (L4, L5, S1)

Arterial supply

Superior gluteal and deep femoral arteries

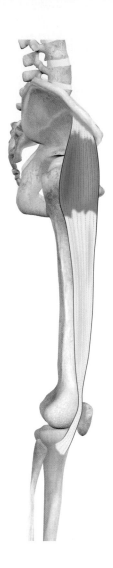

Clinical facts

Works together as synergist with gluteus medius and minimus and the upper fibers of gluteus maximus.

It can often be clearly seen when sprinters are positioned on the starting blocks ready to run.

It is used for sitting, running, cycling, squatting, and in side-kicking movements such as karate.

It has a tendency to cramp if contracted for too long.

A weak tensor fasciae latae may cause the thigh to laterally rotate and the leg may tend to bow. The pelvis will tilt upward on the weak side.

The fascia lata is a tough sheet of connective tissue that serves to divide the thigh into different anatomical compartments: anterior, posterior, medial, lateral.

The tensor fasciae latae (TFL) and the gluteus maximus have a common insertional point in the ITB. The ITB connects the pelvis to the knee and inserts into Gerdy's tubercle on the tibia.

The fiber pattern of TFL mimics that of the deltoid muscle and is often used in reconstructive surgery of the deltoid.

Palpation

1. Performed supine.

2. Place palpating hand along the fibers of tensor fasciae latae; posterior and inferior to the ASIS and anterior aspect of the iliac crest.

3. Instruct patient to actively internally rotate the hip so the contraction of the TFL will feel like an oval mound.

4. Remember to palpate from origin to insertional junction at the ITB.

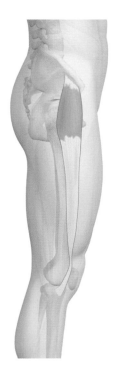

Manual muscle test

Position

Supine, with hip flexed to 60°, abducted 25° and internally rotated.

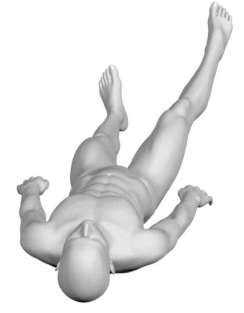

Test

Examiner's resistance is applied diagonally toward opposite ankle (i.e. adduction and slight extension of the hip).
Remember to instruct the client to match and resist the force being applied.
Use an appropriate grading scale to record the findings. Remember to test through the range.
A midrange test can be used to assess isometric strength, wherein the client is instructed to hold the position without a resistant force being applied by the examiner.

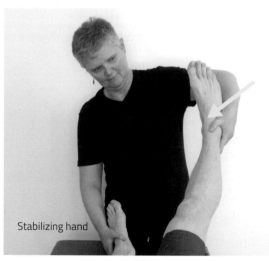

Stabilizing hand

Stabilization

Stabilization can be maintained by examiner placing a hand over the opposite ankle.

Kinesiology muscle test

Position

Supine, with hip flexed to 60°, abducted 25° and internally rotated.

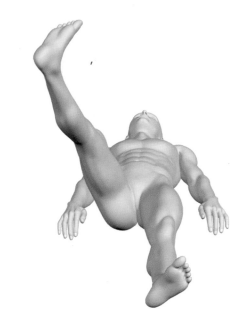

Test

Examiner lightly holds the calcaneus, encouraging internal rotation of the femur. Client is instructed to hold this position whilst the examiner rocks their own body slightly, exerting a light force on the foot. Testing direction is to return the leg toward the couch whilst medially rotating the leg.

Stabilization

Examiner can place the edge of a hand on the opposite thigh or ASIS.

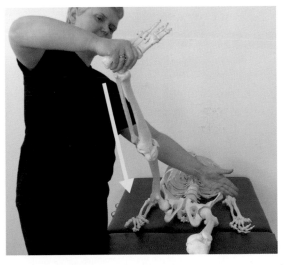

Kinesiological associations

Organ: Large intestine (Note: a bilaterally weak TFL may be found in iron deficiency which should be confirmed by a clinician)
Acupuncture meridian: Large intestine
Emotion: Melancholy, sadness, grief

Video: Tensor fasciae latae

QUADRICEPS FEMORIS GROUP

The quadriceps femoris group is a composite of four muscles, namely: rectus femoris, vastus medialis, vastus intermedius, and vastus lateralis. Each of these muscles will be dealt with separately but they can be tested as a group by kinesiology muscle testing.

Origin

Rectus femoris
Anterior inferior iliac spine (AIIS)
Vastus medialis
Medial lip of linea aspera of femur
Vastus lateralis
Lateral lip of linea aspera, gluteal tuberosity and greater trochanter of femur
Vastus intermedius
Anterior and lateral shaft of femur

Insertion

Via patella and patellar ligament (quadriceps tendon) to tibial tuberosity

Action

All
Extension of knee (tibiofemoral joint)
Helps to control knee flexion when eccentrically contracted
Rectus femoris
Flexion of hip (femoral or coxal joint)

Nerve supply

Femoral nerve
L2, L3, L4

Arterial supply

Femoral artery

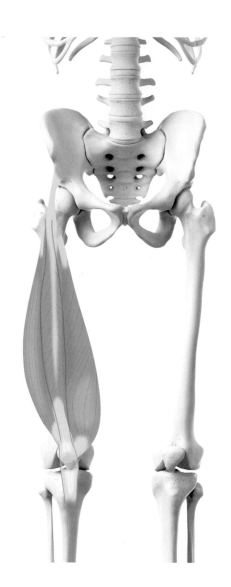

Clinical facts

Quadriceps femoris are used as an anti-gravity muscle when sitting and rising to stand. Synergists include psoas major and minor and sartorius; antagonists include the hamstring group.

They are used to walk, to climb stairs, and to squat. Footballers have well developed quadriceps as they use them during the kicking action of flexing the hip and extending the knee.

Quadriceps group are implicated in patellofemoral syndrome and Osgood–Schlatter's disease.

Palpation

1. Supine. Ask client to extend knee and fully contract the quadriceps group.
2. Look for the shaping of quadriceps muscles.
3. Palpate distal ends of vastus medialis and vastus lateralis.
4. Observe and palpate movement at patella during knee extension.

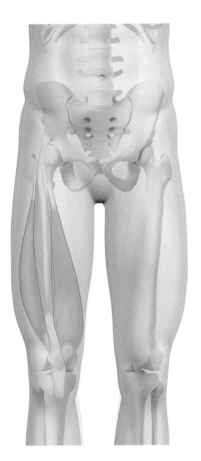

Manual muscle test

Position

As explained above, the group is a composite of four muscles and works to extend the knee, with some muscles acting as hip flexors. To test the group, instruct the client to lie supine with knee and hip flexed to 90°.

Test

Examiner applies a resistance force toward hip and knee extension.

Stabilization

The examiner places their hand over the client's distal thigh and instructs client to grip the treatment couch with their hand.

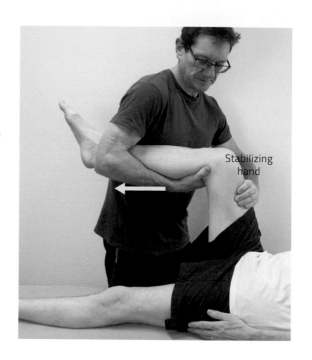

Stabilizing hand

Kinesiology muscle test

Position

Seated, so hip is already flexed. Client extends the knee but does not lock the knee straight.

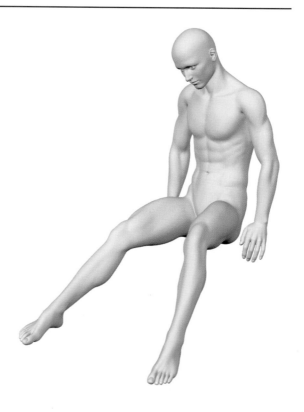

Test

Client is instructed to hold this position. Practitioner rocks their own body slightly, exerting a light pressure on the distal tibia as if to flex the knee.

Stabilization

Support the posterior femur with a hand to lift the leg slightly away from edge of the treatment couch.

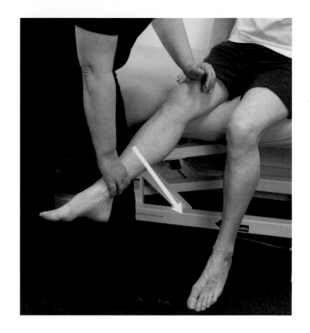

Kinesiological associations

Organ: Small intestine
Acupuncture meridian: Small intestine
Emotion: Worry

Video: Quadriceps femoris group

RECTUS FEMORIS

Origin

Anterior inferior iliac spine (AIIS) and supra-acetabular groove. Rectus femoris has two heads: an anterior and a posterior

Insertion

Tibial tuberosity (via common quadriceps tendon and patellar ligament)

Action

Extension of knee
Flexion of hip
Helps to control knee flexion and hip extension when eccentrically contracted

Nerve supply

Femoral nerve
L2, L3, L4

Arterial supply

Femoral artery

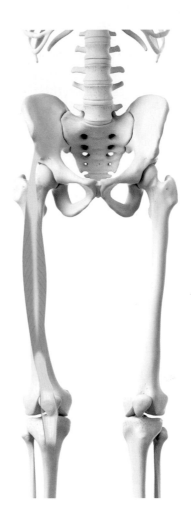

Clinical facts

Works synergistically with vastus intermedius, vastus lateralis, and vastus medialis for knee extension, and iliopsoas, pectineus, and sartorius for hip flexion. Rectus femoris is the only quadriceps muscle to span and act across two joints.

The quadriceps group, together with the gluteus maximus, are anti-gravity muscles. They play an important role in moving from a sitting to a standing position.

Palpation

1. Client is supine or could be seated.
2. Place palpating fingers along fibers just above the patella.
3. Instruct the client to extend the knee.
4. Note the contraction within the muscle tissue. Remember to palpate from origin to insertion.

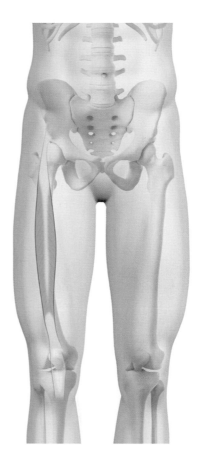

Manual muscle test

Position

Supine. Both hip and knee are flexed to 90°.

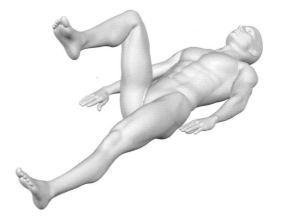

Test

Examiner applies a resistance force toward hip and knee extension.

Use an appropriate grading scale to record the findings. Remember to test through the range.

A midrange test can be used to assess isometric strength, wherein the client is instructed to hold the position without a resistant force being applied by the examiner.

Stabilization

Examiner can stabilize the movement by placing a supporting hand on the client's distal thigh and instructing the client to grip the treatment couch with their hand.

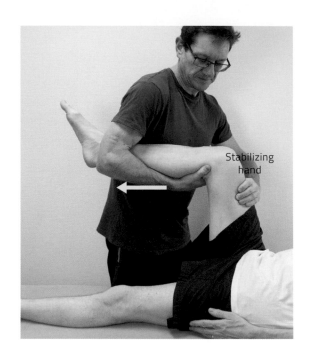

Stabilizing hand

Kinesiology muscle test

Position

Supine. Hip and knee are flexed to 85°.

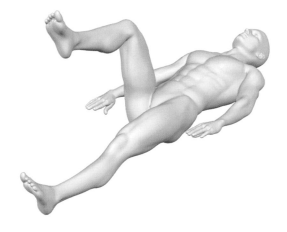

Test

Client is instructed to hold this position. Examiner rocks their body slightly, putting a light pressure on the distal femur, just above the knee, as if bringing the hip and knee into extension.

Stabilization

Support the ankle of the side being tested to keep it at the same height throughout the test.

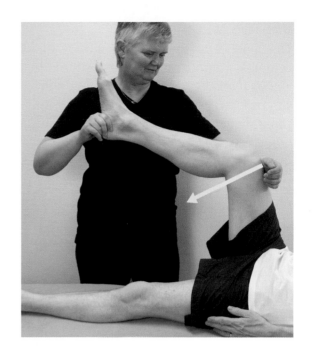

Kinesiological associations

Organ: Small intestine
Acupuncture meridian: Small intestine
Emotion: Worry

Video: Rectus femoris

VASTUS MEDIALIS

The quadriceps femoris group is a composite of four muscles: rectus femoris, vastus medialis, vastus intermedius, and vastus lateralis. Each muscle is dealt with separately but they can be tested as a group by kinesiology muscle testing.

Origin

Medial lip of linea aspera of femur (intertrochanteric line)

Insertion

Via patella and patellar ligament (quadriceps tendon) to tibial tuberosity

Action

Extension of knee (tibiofemoral joint)
Helps to control knee flexion when eccentrically contracted

Nerve supply

Femoral nerve
L2, L3, L4

Arterial supply

Femoral artery

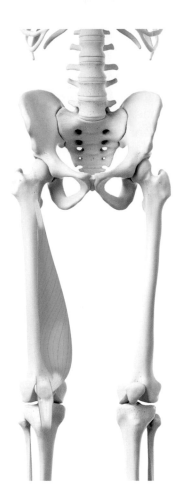

Clinical facts

Works synergistically with vastus intermedius, vastus lateralis, and rectus femoris. The distal fibers of vastus medialis run obliquely at the patella creating a subdivision of the vastus medialis known as the vastus medialis oblique or VMO. The VMO is important in patella tracking. Following patella malalignments of injuries, it is important to strengthen the VMO to ensure optimal function of the knee.

Palpation

1. Supine or seated.
2. Place palpating hand over medial thigh.
3. Ask client to extend knee.
4. Note contraction within vastus medialis, the belly forming a "tear drop shape" at its distal end. Remember to palpate from origin to insertion.

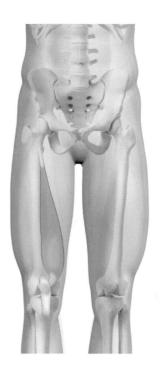

Manual muscle test

Position

Seated with knee partially flexed (15–20°), with lateral rotation of the tibia.

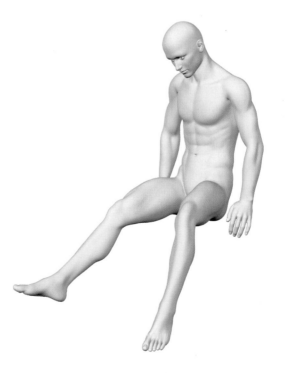

Test

Examiner applies a resistance force toward knee flexion.

Use an appropriate grading scale to record the findings. Remember to test through the range.

A midrange test can be used to assess isometric strength, wherein the client is instructed to hold the position without a resistant force being applied by the examiner.

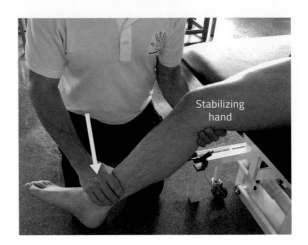

Stabilizing hand

Stabilization

Stabilize the movement by placing a supporting hand on the client's posterior knee, being careful to palpate the soft tissue structures.

Kinesiology muscle test

Not differentiated from quadriceps "group."

Video: Vastus medialis

VASTUS LATERALIS

The quadriceps femoris group is a composite of four muscles: rectus femoris, vastus medialis, vastus intermedius, and vastus lateralis. Each muscle is dealt with separately but they can be tested as a group by kinesiology muscle testing.

Origin

Lateral lip of linea aspera of femur (intertrochanteric line), gluteal tuberosity, and great trochanter

Insertion

Via patella and patellar ligament (quadriceps tendon) to tibial tuberosity

Action

Extension of knee (tibiofemoral joint)
Helps to control knee flexion when eccentrically contracted

Nerve supply

Femoral nerve
L2, L3, L4

Arterial supply

Femoral artery

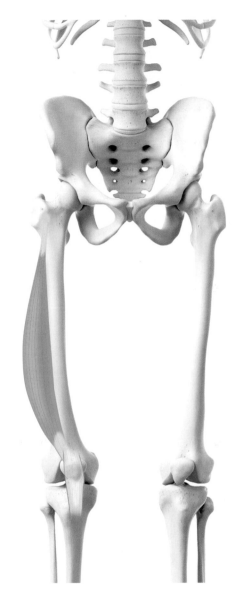

Clinical facts

Works synergistically with vastus intermedius, vastus medialis, and rectus femoris.

This is the largest of the quadriceps muscles. Tightness within the muscle may result in pain referring through the iliotibial band.

Palpation

1. Supine or seated.
2. Place palpating hand over lateral thigh.
3. Ask client to extend knee.
4. Note contraction within vastus lateralis. Remember to palpate from origin to insertion.

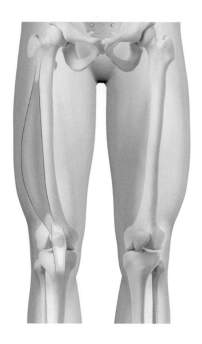

Manual muscle test

Position

Seated with knee partially flexed (30–40°), with medial rotation of the tibia.

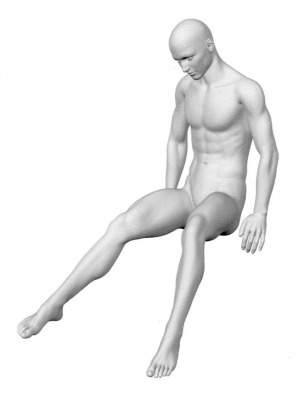

Test

Examiner applies a resistance force toward knee flexion.

Use an appropriate grading scale to record the findings. Remember to test through the range.

A midrange test can be used to assess isometric strength, wherein the client is instructed to hold the position without a resistant force being applied by the examiner.

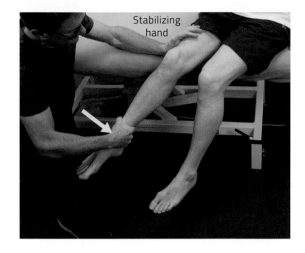

Stabilizing hand

Stabilization

Stabilize the movement by placing a supporting hand on the client's posterior knee, being careful to palpate the soft tissue structures.

Kinesiology muscle test

Not differentiated from quadriceps "group."

Video: Vastus lateralis

VASTUS INTERMEDIUS

The quadriceps femoris group is a composite of four muscles: rectus femoris, vastus medialis, vastus intermedius, and vastus lateralis. Each muscle is dealt with separately but they can be tested as a group by kinesiology muscle testing.

Origin

Anterior lateral femoral surface

Insertion

Via patella and patellar ligament (quadriceps tendon) to tibial tuberosity

Action

Extension of knee (tibiofemoral joint)
Helps to control knee flexion when eccentrically contracted

Nerve supply

Femoral nerve
L2, L3, L4

Arterial supply

Femoral artery

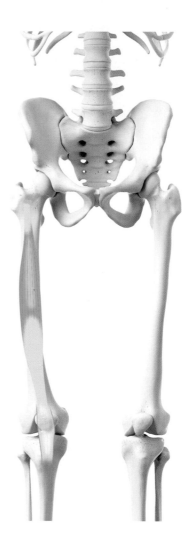

Clinical facts

Works synergistically with vastus medialis, vastus lateralis, and rectus femoris. Vastus intermedius lies deep to the rectus femoris muscle. The lower fibers of vastus intermedius may often blend with the fibers of vastus medialis and lateralis. The distal fibers of the vastus intermedius cover the articularis genu muscle which functions to pull the knee capsule out of extension.

Palpation

1. Supine or seated.
2. Place palpating fingers across the fibers just above the patella.
3. Instruct the client to extend the knee, remembering to palpate deep to the rectus femoris.
4. Note the contraction within the muscle tissue. Remember to palpate from origin to insertion.

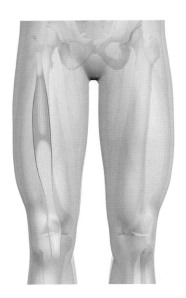

Manual muscle test

Position

Supine with both hip and knee flexed to 90°.

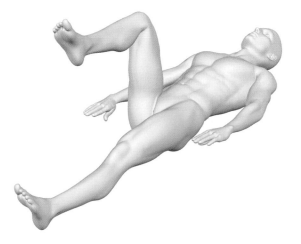

Test

Examiner applies a resistance force toward knee flexion.

Use an appropriate grading scale to record the findings. Remember to test through the range.

A midrange test can be used to assess isometric strength, wherein the client is instructed to hold the position without a resistant force being applied by the examiner.

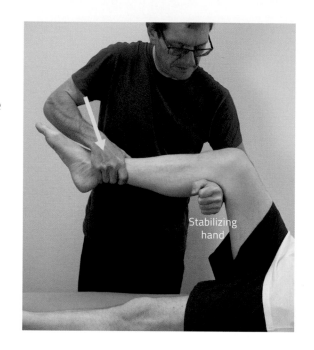

Stabilizing hand

Stabilization

Stabilize the movement by placing a supporting hand on the client's posterior knee, being careful to palpate the soft tissue structures.

Kinesiology muscle test

Not differentiated from quadriceps "group."

Video: Vastus intermedius

HAMSTRING GROUP

Origin

Biceps femoris
Long head: Ischial tuberosity
Short head: Lateral lip of linea aspera
Semitendinosus and semimembranosus
Ischial tuberosity

Insertion

Biceps femoris
Fibula head
Semitendinosus
Proximal anteromedial tibia at pes anserinus
Semimembranosus
Medial condyle of tibia

Action

All
Flexion of knee
Extension of hip
Helps to control knee extension and hip flexion when eccentrically contracted
Biceps femoris
Assists with external rotation of tibia when knee is flexed
Semitendinosus and semimembranosus
Assists with internal rotation of tibia when knee is flexed

Nerve supply

Sciatic nerve complex (tibial branch)
L4, L5, S1, S2

Arterial supply

Inferior gluteal and deep femoral arteries

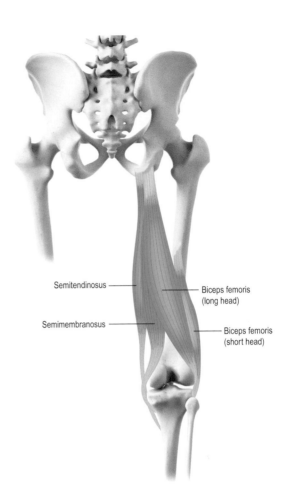

Semitendinosus

Semimembranosus

Biceps femoris (long head)

Biceps femoris (short head)

Clinical facts

The hamstring group is a composite of three main muscles: biceps femoris, semitendinosus, and semimembranosus. The group is named because in medieval times, butchers typically used the hamstring tendons to hang their hams and pig carcasses in the butcher's shop.

The hamstring group are strong hip extensors and knee flexors.
An "anti-gravity" set of muscles, they are used when cycling, running, climbing stairs, and lowering oneself into a chair.
Some anatomists suggest that the fibers of adductor magnus constitute the fourth hamstring.

Palpation

1. Prone. Examiner places hand in the center of posterior thigh and asks client to flex the knee, as if to lift the foot from the treatment couch.
2. Feel for strong contraction of hamstring group.
3. Palpate ischial tuberosity. Move palpating hand slightly below ischial tuberosity to locate hamstring tendons.
4. Palpate from origin to insertion.

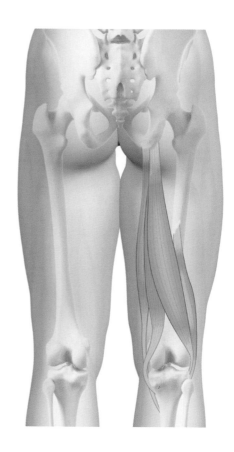

Manual muscle test

Position

The muscle group is a composite of three key muscles as described above. The main action of the group is flexion of the knee and extension of the hip. When testing the group, the client is placed prone, with knee flexed to 90° and hip slightly extended.

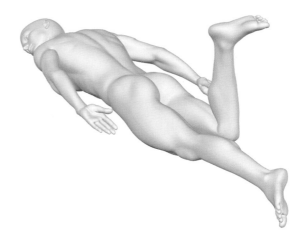

Test

The examiner applies a resistance force toward knee extension.

Stabilization

The stabilizing hand is placed over the lumbar spine and sacral area.

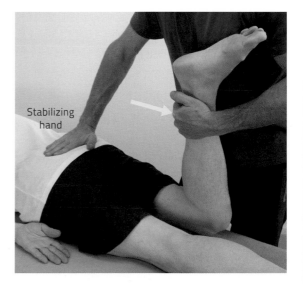

Stabilizing hand

Kinesiology muscle test

Position

Prone, with knee flexed to 70–80°. Keep foot and ankle relaxed to prevent gastrocnemius and soleus involvement.

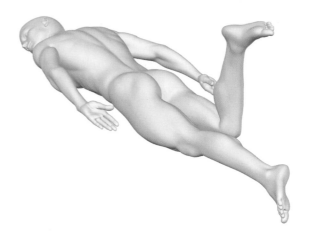

Test

Client is asked to hold this position. Practitioner stands beside client's lower leg, facing up the body, and holds the distal tibia. Practitioner gently rocks their own body backward, exerting a light pressure on the distal tibia, as if extending the knee.

Stabilization

Apply a reasonable amount of pressure on the hamstrings using a clenched fist into the belly of the muscles. This prevents cramping of the hamstrings.

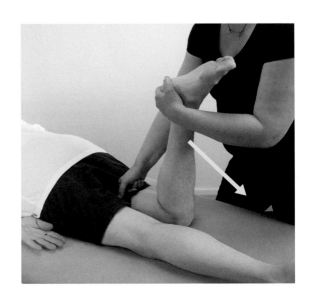

Kinesiological associations

Organ: Large intestine, rectum
Acupuncture meridian: Large intestine
Emotion: Sadness

Video: Hamstring group

BICEPS FEMORIS

Origin

Long head
Ischial tuberosity
Short head
Lateral lip of linea aspera of femur

Insertion

Fibula head

Action

Flexion of knee
Extension of hip
Further assists with external tibial rotation
(lateral) when knee is flexed (long head only)
Helps to control knee extension and hip
flexion when eccentrically contracted

Nerve supply

Long head
Sciatic nerve – tibial branch
L5, S1, S2, S3
Short head
Sciatic nerve – common peroneal division
L5, S1, S2

Arterial supply

Long head
Inferior gluteal and deep femoral arteries
Short head
Deep femoral artery

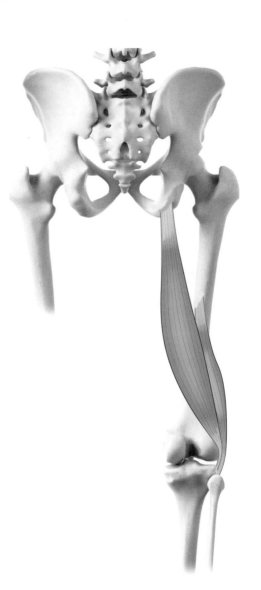

Clinical facts

Works synergistically with semitendinosus and semimembranosus to produce knee flexion and hip extension.

Biceps femoris further works synergistically with gastrocnemius, gracilis, and sartorius to produce knee flexion.

The short head is occasionally absent. This muscle is commonly referred to as the lateral hamstring and is the only hamstring muscle which has two heads.

Palpation

1. Performed prone.
2. Place palpating fingers along fiber direction of biceps femoris just below the ischial tuberosity.
3. Instruct the client to flex the knee.
4. Note the contraction within the muscle tissue. Remember to palpate from origin to insertion.

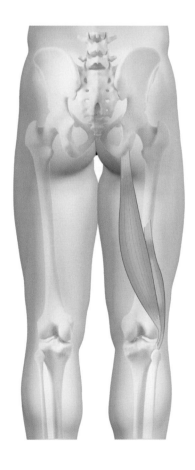

Manual muscle test

Position

Prone, with knee flexed to 85°, hip slightly adducted and laterally rotated.

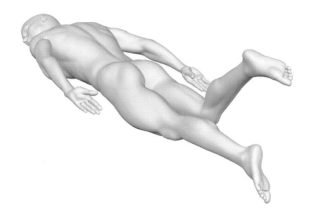

Test

Examiner applies a resistance force toward knee extension.

Use an appropriate grading scale to record the findings. Remember to test through the range.

A midrange test can be used to assess isometric strength, wherein the client is instructed to hold the position without a resistant force being applied by the examiner.

Stabilization

Place a stabilizing hand on client's sacrum.

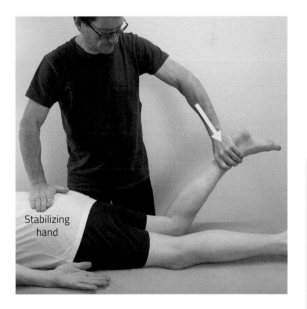

Stabilizing hand

Kinesiology muscle test

Position

Prone, with knee flexed to 85°. Observe posterior thigh to note the direction of pressure needed to cause some contraction of biceps femoris without putting tension on medial hamstrings (semimembranosus and semitendinosus). Keep foot and ankle in neutral, to prevent contraction of soleus and gastrocnemius.

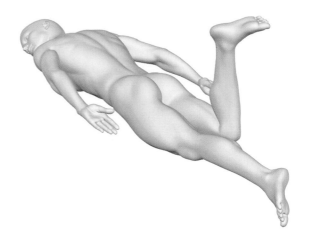

Test

Client is asked to hold this position. Practitioner stands beside client's lower leg, facing up the body, and holds the distal tibia. Practitioner gently rocks their own body backward, exerting a light pressure on the distal tibia, as if extending the knee.

Stabilization

Apply a reasonable amount of pressure on the hamstrings using a clenched fist into the belly of the muscles. This prevents cramping of the hamstrings.

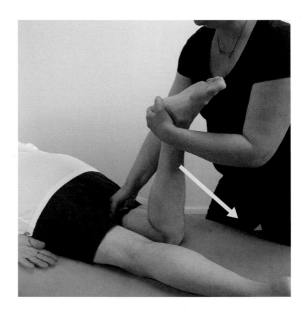

Kinesiological associations

Organ: Large intestine
Acupuncture meridian: Large intestine
Emotion: Sadness

Video: Biceps femoris

MEDIAL HAMSTRINGS (semitendinosus and semimembranosus)

Origin

Semitendinosus
Ischial tuberosity
Semimembranosus
Ischial tuberosity

Insertion

Semitendinosus
Proximal, medial shaft of tibia at pes anserinus tendon
Semimembranosus
Posterior, medial condyle of tibia

Action

Flexion of knee (tibiofemoral joint)
Medial rotation (internal) of flexed knee (tibiofemoral joint)
Extension of hip (femoral or coxal joint)

Nerve supply

Sciatic nerve complex (tibial branch)
L4, L5, S1, S2

Arterial supply

Inferior gluteal and deep femoral arteries

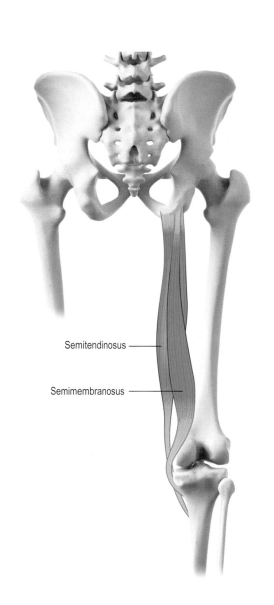

Semitendinosus

Semimembranosus

Clinical facts

Semitendinosus and semimembranosus are collectively known as the medial hamstring; this is the largest of the hamstring muscles.

Both semitendinosus and semimembranosus work synergistically with biceps femoris to produce knee flexion and hip extension. They work synergistically with gastrocnemius, gracilis, and sartorius to aid knee flexion.

The proximal fibers of semitendinosus may blend with the fibers of the long head of biceps femoris. It is often divided into a superior and inferior portion through an oblique tendinous intersection within the muscle belly. The insertion of semitendinosus into the pes anserinus acts as an attachment point for the sartorius and gracilis.

Distal fibers of semimembranosus blend with proximal fibers of gastrocnemius. Distal fibers also fan out and attach to medial meniscus of knee, where it functions to pull medial meniscus posteriorly, thus preventing meniscus impingement.

Palpation

1. Performed prone.
2. Place palpating fingers along fiber direction just below the ischial tuberosity.
3. Instruct the client to flex the knee against resistance.
4. Note the contraction within the muscle tissue. Remember to palpate from origin to insertion.

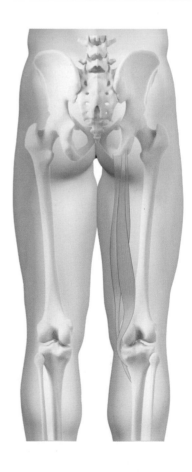

Manual muscle test

Semitendinosus and semimembranosus manual muscle tests are performed as a group test for medial hamstrings.

Position

Prone, with knee flexed to 85° and hip slightly abducted and knee medially rotated.

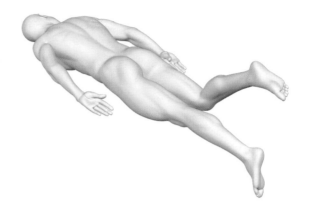

Test

Examiner applies a resistance force toward knee extension.

Use an appropriate grading scale to record the findings. Remember to test through the range.

A midrange test can be used to assess isometric strength, wherein the client is instructed to hold the position without a resistant force being applied by the examiner.

Stabilization

Examiner can stabilize the movement by placing a supporting hand on the client's sacrum.

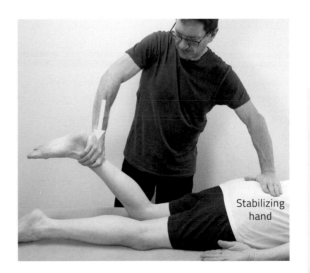

Stabilizing hand

Kinesiology muscle test

Semitendinosus and semimembranosus kinesiology muscle tests are performed as a group test for medial hamstrings.

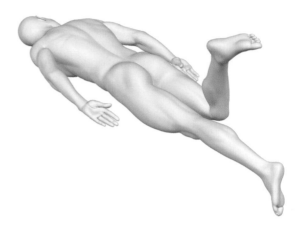

Position

Prone, with knee flexed to 70–80° with slight medial rotation. Observe posterior thigh to note the direction of pressure needed to cause some contraction of medial hamstrings without putting tension on biceps femoris. Keep foot and ankle relaxed to prevent gastrocnemius and soleus involvement.

Test

Client is asked to hold this position. Practitioner stands beside client's lower leg, facing up the body, and holds the distal tibia. Practitioner gently rocks their own body backward, exerting a light pressure on the distal tibia, as if extending the knee.

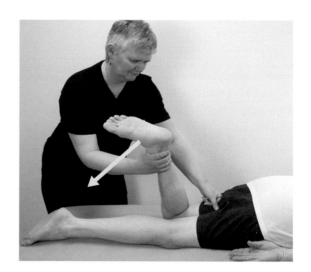

Stabilization

Apply a reasonable amount of pressure on the hamstrings using a clenched fist into the belly of the muscles. This prevents cramping of the hamstrings and allows palpation of the medial hamstrings as they contract.

Kinesiological associations

Organ: Large intestine
Acupuncture meridian: Large intestine
Emotion: Sadness

Video: Medial hamstrings

ADDUCTOR MAGNUS

Origin
Anterior head
Inferior pubic ramus and ischial ramus
Posterior head
Ischial tuberosity

Insertion
Anterior head
Medial lip of linea aspera of the femur
Posterior head
Adductor tubercle just proximal to the
medial femoral epicondyle

Action
Adduction and extension of the hip
(femoral/coxal joint)
The anterior head assists with lateral
rotation of the thigh
Helps to control abduction of the hip when
eccentrically contracted
Helps to stabilize pelvis when walking

Nerve supply
Anterior head
Obturator nerve
L2, L3, L4
Posterior head
Sciatic nerve complex (tibial branch)
L4, L5, S1

Arterial supply
Femoral and deep femoral arteries

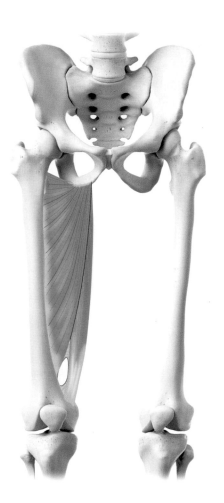

Clinical facts

Works synergistically with biceps femoris, semimembranosus, and semitendinosus to produce hip extension. It also works synergistically with adductor brevis and longus, pectineus, gracilis to aid hip adduction. Adductor magnus is divided into two compartments through an anterior and posterior head. The anterior head is the adductor component, whereas the posterior head works synergistically with the hamstring group.

Interestingly, the anterior head can further be divided into a superior part with horizontal fiber arrangements called "adductor minimus" and a middle section with more oblique fibers. Some clinicians classify the "adductor minimus" as its own muscle. Adductor magnus may be considered as the fourth hamstring muscle, because of its posterior attachment and action.

Palpation

1. Performed prone or side lying.
2. Place palpating fingers along fiber direction just below the ischial tuberosity.
3. Instruct the client to adduct the hip against resistance.
4. Note the contraction within the muscle tissue. Remember to palpate from origin to insertion.
5. Note this muscle can also be palpated with the client in a supine position, by palpating posteriorly to gracilis.

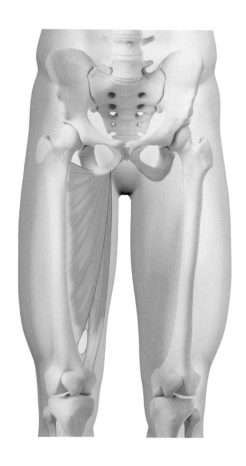

Manual muscle test

Position

Supine with hip flexed 8–15° and medially (internally) rotated.

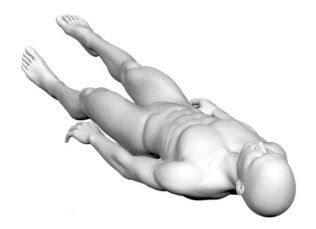

Test

Examiner applies a resistance force diagonally toward abduction and flexion. Use an appropriate grading scale to record the findings. Remember to test through the range.
A midrange test can be used to assess isometric strength, wherein the client is instructed to hold the position without a resistant force being applied by the examiner.

Stabilization

Place a supporting hand on the client's opposite lower leg or ankle.

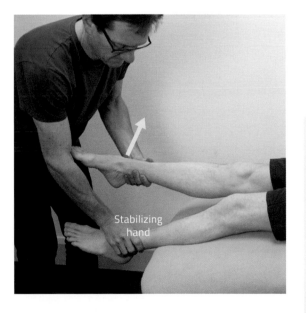

Stabilizing hand

Kinesiology muscle test

Position

Supine. Adduct legs together with slight medial (internal) rotation to the leg being tested.

This test can be disorientating for the client, as to which leg is being tested. To prevent recruitment of the contralateral adductors, squeeze the distal portion of the leg being tested just prior to the test, so client knows which one to hold in position.

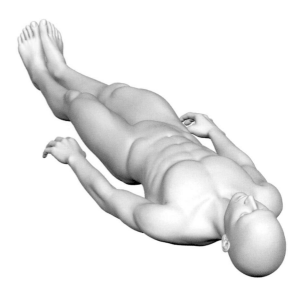

Test

Client is instructed to hold this position. Practitioner stands beside the leg being tested, holding the distal part of lower leg. Practitioner rocks their own body slightly, exerting a gentle pressure on the medial surface of lower leg, as if to abduct the leg.

Stabilization

Hold the distal tibia of non-tested leg.

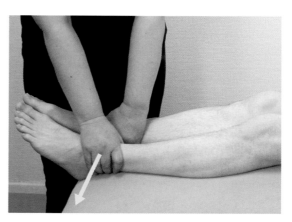

Kinesiological associations

Organ: Reproductive and endocrine organs including thyroid, pituitary, and adrenal (particularly in menopause or change in endocrine function)
Acupuncture meridian: Circulation/sex
Emotion: Various, depending on associated organ

Video: Adductor magnus

ADDUCTOR LONGUS AND BREVIS

Origin

Adductor longus
Anterior pubic surface
Adductor brevis
Body and inferior ramus of pubis

Insertion

Medial lip of linea aspera (adductor longus attaches at roughly middle third, whereas adductor brevis has the same insertion occupying the proximal third) and pectineal line

Action

Adduction and flexion of hip (femoral/coxal joint)
Lateral rotation of thigh
Helps to control abduction of the hip when eccentrically loaded
Helps to stabilize the pelvis when walking

Nerve supply

Obturator nerve
L2, L3, L4

Arterial supply

Femoral and obturator arteries

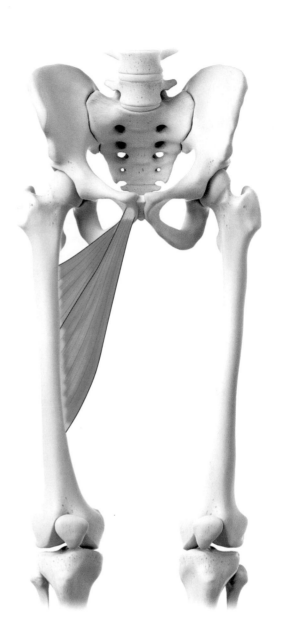

Clinical facts

Works synergistically with adductor magnus, pectineus, gracilis to aid hip adduction and flexion.

Distal fibers of adductor longus often join with those of vastus medialis near the linea aspera.

The groin is a crowded region for multiple muscle attachments, so attachments of the adductors within the groin makes it often difficult to isolate each muscle in turn. Adductor longus is, however, the most prominent tendon in the groin, and can be palpated on the medial aspect of the groin. A "pulled groin" often refers to an injury within the adductor longus and/or brevis. In sport, Gilmore's groin is synonymous with an adductor tear and is typically considered to be a sportsman's hernia, despite no herniated tissue being present.

Palpation

1. Client is supine.

2. Place palpating fingers along fiber direction over medial upper thigh.

3. Instruct the client to adduct the hip against resistance.

4. Note the contraction within the muscle tissue. Remember to palpate from origin to insertion.

5. To differentiate adductor brevis from longus, palpate lateral and often deep to adductor longus.

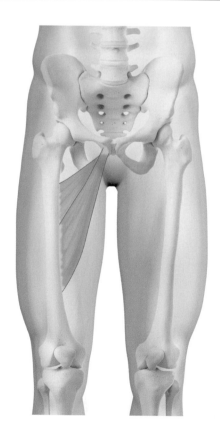

Manual muscle test

Position

Supine, with hip flexed 20–30° and medially (internally) rotated.

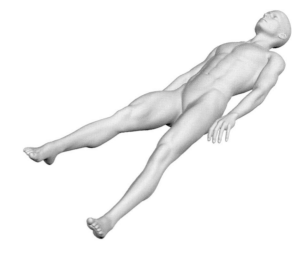

Test

Examiner applies a resistance force diagonally toward hip abduction.
Use an appropriate grading scale to record the findings. Remember to test through the range.
A midrange test can be used to assess isometric strength, wherein the client is instructed to hold the position without a resistant force being applied by the examiner.

Stabilization

Place a supporting hand on the client's opposite lower leg or ankle.

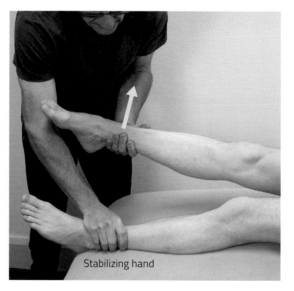

Stabilizing hand

Kinesiology muscle test

Not performed.

Video: Adductor longus and brevis

GRACILIS

Origin
Inferior ramus and body of pubis

Insertion
Proximal anterior medial aspect of tibia (pes anserinus)

Action
Adduction of the hip
Internal (medial) rotation of the flexed knee

Nerve supply
Obturator nerve
L2, L3, L4

Arterial supply
Femoral and obturator arteries

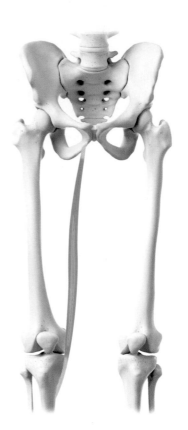

Clinical facts

Works synergistically with adductor magnus, longus/brevis and pectineus to aid hip adduction.
This is the most medial thigh muscle and second longest in the body next to sartorius. Gracilis acts across two joints (hip and knee). Surgically, gracilis is the muscle often used in upper and lower limb reconstruction procedures.

Palpation

1. Client is supine with knee flexed, hip slightly flexed and laterally rotated.
2. Place palpating fingers along fiber direction over medial thigh.
3. Instruct the client to adduct the hip.
4. Note the contraction within the muscle tissue. Remember to palpate from origin to insertion.

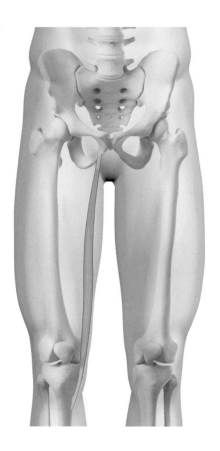

Manual muscle test

Position

Supine with hip medially rotated.

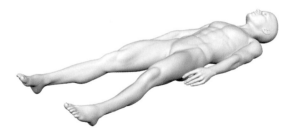

Test

Examiner applies a resistance force toward hip abduction.

Use an appropriate grading scale to record the findings. Remember to test through the range.

A midrange test can be used to assess isometric strength, wherein the client is instructed to hold the position without a resistant force being applied by the examiner.

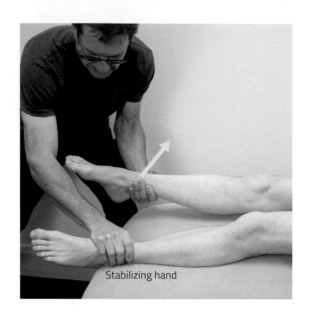

Stabilizing hand

Stabilization

Examiner can stabilize the movement by placing a supporting hand on the client's opposite lower leg or ankle.

Kinesiology muscle test

Position

Prone. Client flexes the knee to approximately 45° with hip internally (medially) rotated by bringing foot laterally. Bring hip into slight extension by lifting the knee from the treatment couch.

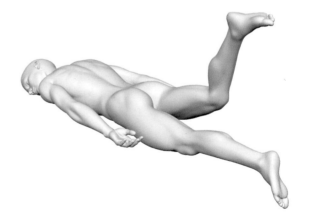

Test

Client is instructed to hold this position. Examiner rocks their own body slightly, exerting light pressure on medial surface of distal tibia, as if to extend the knee with slight medial hip rotation.

Stabilization

Leg can be lifted onto examiner's thigh or supported under the knee.

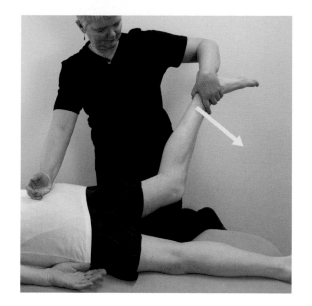

Kinesiological associations

Organ: Adrenals
Acupuncture meridian: Circulation/sex and triple warmer
Emotion: Stress and anxiety

Video: Gracilis

POPLITEUS

Origin
Lateral condyle of femur

Insertion
Proximal posterior tibia, medial aspect of soleal line

Action
Helps to unlock the knee from an extended position
Helps external (lateral) rotation of the femur on the tibia
Helps internal (medial) rotation of the tibia on the femur and flexion of the knee

Nerve supply
Tibial nerve
L4, L5, S1

Arterial supply
Popliteal artery

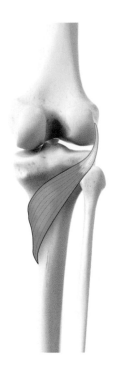

Clinical facts

Works synergistically with gastrocnemius, semitendinosus, semimembranosus, and biceps femoris (hamstring group). Popliteus helps to stabilize the knee posteriorly and is nicknamed "the key that unlocks the knee" as it initiates knee flexion by laterally rotating the femur on the tibia. Popliteus is the deepest of the muscles at the posterior of the knee. It has fibers which attach to the lateral meniscus which pull the lateral meniscus posteriorly during knee flexion. This helps to prevent impingement of the meniscus. It is often implicated in posterior knee pain when running, especially downhill, and can be damaged by stop-start running actions, skiing accidents, and twisting injuries in football or rugby. The proximal tendon of popliteus cross through the lateral capsule of the knee and can be involved in posterior cruciate ligament injuries.

Palpation

1. Client is seated or prone with knee flexed between 40° and 80°.

2. Place palpating fingers over fibers on the posterior knee and locate both the origin and insertion of the muscle.

3. Instruct the client to internally rotate the tibia. Because of its depth, it is hard to palpate the belly of the muscle, but its insertion on the posterior tibia can be palpated.

4. Note the contraction within the muscle tissue. Remember to palpate from origin to insertion, deep to the gastrocnemius.

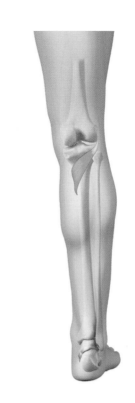

Manual muscle test

Position

Supine with leg extended and internally rotated, knee is partially flexed to 20°.

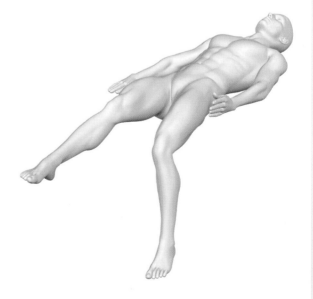

Test

Examiner applies a resistance force toward knee external rotation. Use an appropriate grading scale to record the findings. Remember to test through the range. A midrange test can be used to assess isometric strength, wherein the client is instructed to hold the position without a resistant force being applied by the examiner.

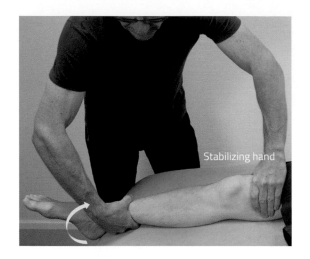

Stabilizing hand

Stabilization

Examiner can stabilize the movement by placing a supporting hand proximal to the patella.

Kinesiology muscle test

Position

Supine. Client flexes knee to 90° and externally rotates hip so knee drops out laterally, supporting the ankle.

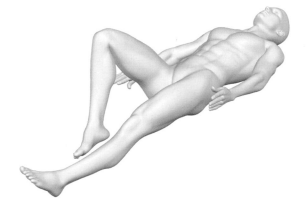

Test

Client is instructed to hold this position. Examiner rocks their body slightly, exerting a light force on the lateral side of the knee whilst holding the ankle so lower leg twists in opposite direction. If popliteus is strong, this torque will be felt and observed in the hip muscles. If weak, no torque is observed and lower leg will easily twist.

Stabilization

Stabilize the ankle so the lower leg can be twisted in opposite direction from femur.

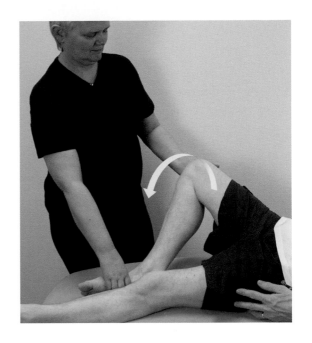

Kinesiological associations

Organ: Gall bladder
Acupuncture meridian: Gall bladder
Emotion: Irritability, frustration

Video: Popliteus

SARTORIUS

Origin

Anterior superior iliac spine (ASIS)

Insertion

Proximal anteromedial aspect of tibia (pes anserinus)

Action

Flexion of hip and knee
Abduction of hip (coxal joint)
External (lateral) rotation of hip and internal (medial) rotation of flexed knee
Assists with initiation of an anterior pelvic tilt

Nerve supply

Femoral nerve
L2, L3, L4

Arterial supply

Femoral artery

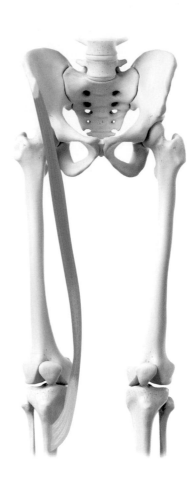

Clinical facts

Works synergistically with gracilis, semitendinosus, semimembranosus, and biceps femoris.
Sartorius is considered the longest muscle in the body and is commonly referred to as the tailor's muscle, named for the action it produces when crossing the legs, the traditional position used by tailors when they are sewing.

Palpation

1. Client is supine. Place leg being palpated across the other leg as if forming a "figure 4" so the foot is resting just below the opposite knee with the hip flexed and slightly laterally (externally) rotated.

2. Place palpating fingers along the fibers just below and medial to the ASIS.

3. Instruct the client to flex and externally rotate the hip.

4. Note the contraction within the muscle tissue in the superficially placed sartorius. Remember to palpate from origin to insertion.

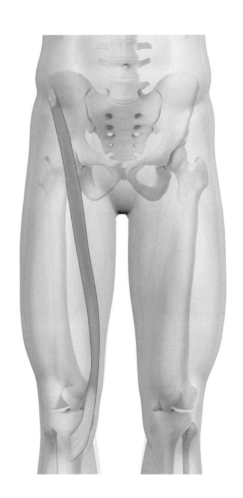

Manual muscle test

Position

Supine, with leg being tested slightly flexed and laterally rotated at hip and slightly flexed at knee, with foot placed just below the opposite patella, such that the leg looks like a number 4.

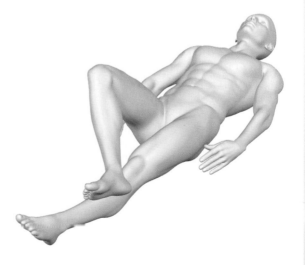

Test

Examiner applies a resistance force toward adduction and internal rotation of the hip as the primary force, or a secondary one could be applied toward knee and hip extension. Use an appropriate grading scale to record the findings. Remember to test through the range.

A midrange test can be used to assess isometric strength, wherein the client is instructed to hold the position without a resistant force being applied by the examiner.

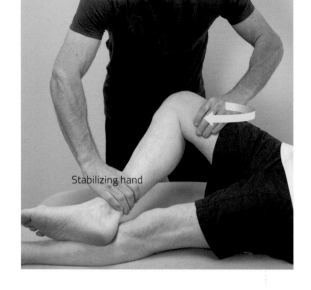

Stabilizing hand

Stabilization

Stabilization occurs by client firmly gripping the side of the treatment couch.

Kinesiology muscle test

Position

Supine, with leg being tested slightly flexed and laterally rotated at hip and slightly flexed at knee, with foot placed just below the opposite patella, such that the leg looks like a number 4.

Examiner weight-bears the test by standing at the end of the couch so the client's uninvolved foot is placed against the examiner's leg.

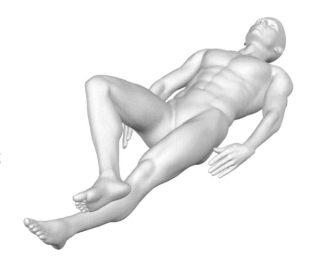

Test

Client is instructed to hold this position, whilst the examiner holds the ankle and rocks their own body slightly, attempting to straighten the knee.

Stabilization

Support is given at the knee to prevent it laterally rotating further. Client can be instructed to place both hands under the occiput during sartorius testing as a form of "double therapy localization."

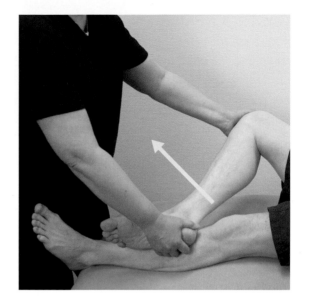

Kinesiological associations

Organ: Adrenals
Acupuncture meridian: Triple warmer and circulation/sex
Emotion: Stress

Video: Sartorius

GASTROCNEMIUS

Together with the soleus and plantaris muscles, the gastrocnemius forms the "triceps surae" group.

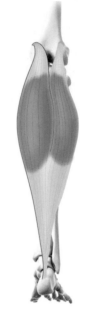

Origin

Medial head
Superior to medial femoral condyle on posterior surface
Lateral head
Superior to lateral femoral condyle on posterior surface

Insertion

Calcaneus via calcaneal tendon (Achilles)

Action

Weakly flexes the knee (tibiofemoral joint)
Plantarflexes the foot at ankle (talocrural joint)
Helps to control dorsiflexion of foot at the ankle when eccentrically contracted

Nerve supply

Tibial nerve
S1, S2

Arterial supply

Sural branch of popliteal artery

Clinical facts

Works synergistically with soleus, plantaris, tibialis posterior, peroneus longus and brevis, flexor hallucis longus, flexor digitorum longus.
Proximal fibers may blend with the posterior portion of the knee capsule.
Gastrocnemius is important in stabilizing the ankle and knee when standing.
Wearing high heels for prolonged periods could result in chronic shortening of the triceps surae.

Sonographic imaging has revealed a sesamoid bone between the lateral head of gastrocnemius and posterior femoral condyle. This is called the fabella.
The Achilles reflex tests spinal nerve S1.
The triceps surae group are important vascular pump muscles which assist venous return to the heart and aid lymphatic return.

Palpation

1. Client is prone with knee extended.
2. Place palpating fingers over fibers on the posterior leg.
3. Instruct the client to plantarflex the foot and ankle.
4. Note the contraction within the muscle tissue. Remember to palpate from origin to insertion.

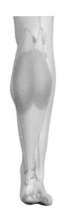

Manual muscle test

Position

Performed supine, with knee and hip flexed to 90° and ankle plantarflexed.

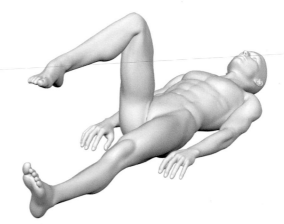

Test

Examiner applies a resistance force by attempting to pull the calcaneus into dorsiflexion.

Use an appropriate grading scale to record the findings. Remember to test through the range. A midrange test can be used to assess isometric strength, wherein the client is instructed to hold the position without a resistant force being applied by the examiner.

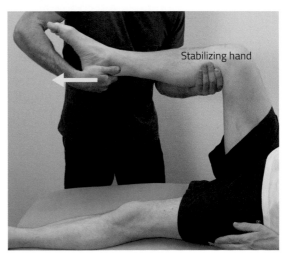

Stabilizing hand

Stabilization

Examiner can stabilize the movement by placing a supporting hand proximal to the posterior knee.

Kinesiology muscle test

Position

Performed supine. Slightly flex the hip and knee with the foot fully plantarflexed. Gastrocnemius lateral and medial portions can be tested by medially rotating the lower leg for testing the medial portion, and laterally rotating the lower leg for lateral portion.

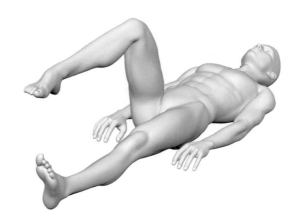

Test

Client is asked to hold this position. Examiner holds the ankle and rocks their own body, exerting a light pressure, and attempts to extend the knee.

Stabilization

Examiner holds the knee during the test to stabilize the leg.

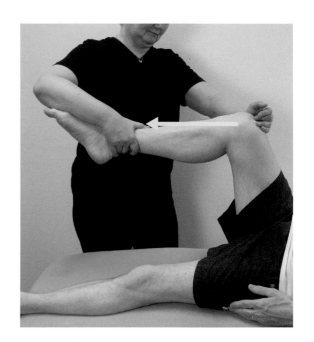

Kinesiological associations

Organ: Adrenal
Acupuncture meridian: Circulation/sex and triple warmer
Emotion: Stress

Video: Gastrocnemius

SOLEUS

Origin
Soleal line of tibia and proximal aspect of head of fibula

Insertion
Calcaneus via the calcaneal tendon (Achilles)

Action
Plantarflexes the foot at the ankle (talocrural joint)
Inverts the foot (weakly)
Helps to control dorsiflexion of the ankle (talocrural joint)

Nerve supply
Tibial nerve
L5, S1, S2

Arterial supply
Sural branch of popliteal artery

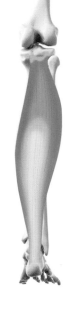

Clinical facts

Works synergistically with gastrocnemius, plantaris, tibialis posterior, peroneus longus and brevis, flexor hallucis longus, flexor digitorum longus.
Soleus is the main plantarflexor of the foot and is important in stabilizing the ankle and knee when standing. It is an important lower limb postural muscle.
Wearing high heels for prolonged periods could result in chronic shortening of the soleus and triceps surae.

Sonographic imaging has revealed an extra belly called the accessory soleus. Sometimes the medial portion of soleus may be shown to be absent.
The Achilles reflex tests spinal nerve S1.
The triceps surae group are important vascular pump muscles whish assist venous return to the heart and lymphatic return.
Soleus is named because of its shape resembling a sole fish.

Palpation

1. Client is prone with knee flexed to 90°.
2. Place palpating fingers over fibers on the posterior leg.
3. Instruct the client to plantarflex the foot and ankle.
4. Note the contraction within the muscle tissue. Remember to palpate from origin to insertion, deep to the gastrocnemius.

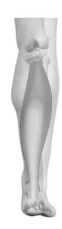

Manual muscle test

Position

Performed prone, with knee flexed to 110° and ankle/foot plantarflexed.

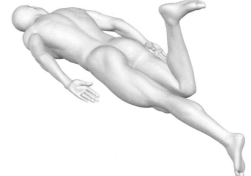

Test

Examiner applies a resistance force by attempting to lift the calcaneus into dorsiflexion.

Use an appropriate grading scale to record the findings. Remember to test through the range.

A midrange test can be used to assess isometric strength, wherein the client is instructed to hold the position without a resistant force being applied by the examiner.

Stabilization

Examiner can stabilize the movement by placing a supportive hand on the proximal tibia.

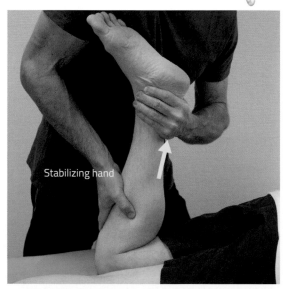

Stabilizing hand

Kinesiology muscle test

Position

Prone. Knee is flexed to just under 90° to remove any involvement of gastrocnemius in the test. Do not flex more than 90° or hamstrings will become involved in this test. Fully plantarflex the foot.

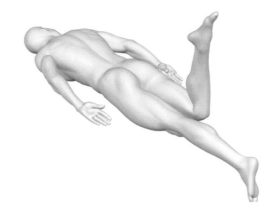

Test

Client is asked to hold this position. Examiner holds the calcaneus. Examiner rocks their body slightly, exerting a light pressure to the calcaneus and plantar surface of foot as if to cause dorsiflexion of the foot.

Stabilization

Examiner places a hand on the plantar surface of the foot and directs the foot into dorsiflexion.

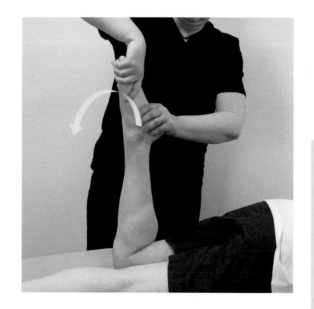

Kinesiological associations

Organ: Adrenal
Acupuncture meridian: Circulation/sex and triple warmer
Emotion: Stress

Video: Soleus

TIBIALIS ANTERIOR

Origin

Proximal lateral two thirds of tibia, lateral condyle of tibia and interosseous membrane

Insertion

Medial cuneiform and base of 1st metatarsal. Anterior tibialis tendon runs anterior to the medial malleolus of tibia

Action

Inversion of foot at subtalar joint
Dorsiflexion of ankle (talocrural joint)
Helps to control eversion of foot at subtalar joint and plantarflexion of the ankle at talocrural joint when eccentrically contracted

Nerve supply

Deep peroneal nerve
L4, L5, S1

Arterial supply

Anterior tibial artery

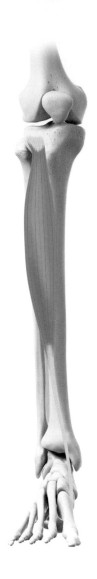

Clinical facts

Works synergistically with extensor hallucis longus, extensor digitorum longus.
Tibialis anterior supports the medial longitudinal arch, particularly in balancing, running, and walking, and helps the swing phase of gait as it lifts the foot so it clears the ground after toe-off.
Tibialis anterior pain can result from tightness and/or damage to the tibialis anterior and lead to shin splints.

Lesions of the deep peroneal nerve can cause paralysis in the tibialis anterior resulting in a dropped foot. Foot drop prevents the heel from striking the ground first, thereby forcing the individual to raise their arch and toes to prevent the toes from hitting the ground. The result is a distinctive clop or foot slapping sound.

Palpation

1. Client is supine or seated.

2. Place palpating fingers over tibialis anterior fibers just lateral to the anterior section of the tibia.

3. Instruct the client to dorsiflex the ankle and curl the toes downward. By flexing the toes in this way, one can eliminate the contracture involvement of extensor digitorum longus.

4. Note the contraction within the muscle tissue. Remember to palpate from origin to insertion.

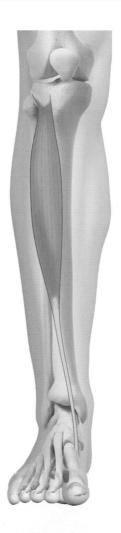

Manual muscle test

Position

Usually performed supine with ankle dorsiflexed and inverted.

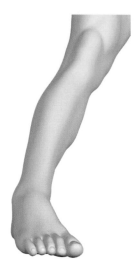

Test

Examiner applies a resistance force on the foot, diagonally from medial to lateral and toward plantarflexion.

Use an appropriate grading scale to record the findings. Remember to test through the range.

A midrange test can be used to assess isometric strength, wherein the client is instructed to hold the position without a resistant force being applied by the examiner.

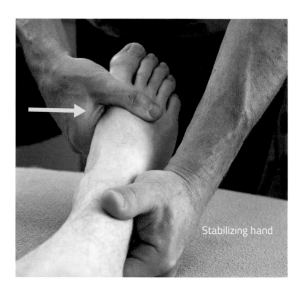

Stabilizing hand

Stabilization

Examiner can stabilize the movement by placing a supporting hand lateral to the ankle.

Kinesiology muscle test

Position

Performed supine. Fully dorsiflex and invert the foot. (UP AND IN)

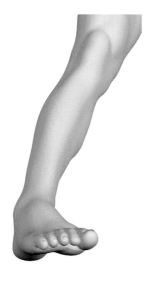

Test

Client is instructed to hold this position. Examiner holds the foot with both hands and moves slightly laterally, exerting a light pressure on the foot as if to bring the foot back into neutral position.

Stabilization

Holding the foot with both hands allows the examiner to move their body easily. Any movement in the client will therefore occur at the ankle.

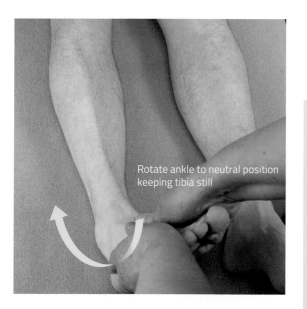

Rotate ankle to neutral position keeping tibia still

Kinesiological associations

Organ: Bladder
Acupuncture meridian: Urinary bladder
Emotion: Fear

Video: Tibialis anterior

TIBIALIS POSTERIOR

Origin

Posterior proximal two thirds of the tibia, fibula, and interosseous membrane

Insertion

Plantar surface of foot including the navicular, all three cuneiforms, 2nd, 3rd, and 4th metatarsals, cuboid and calcaneus. Posterior tibialis tendon runs under the medial malleolus of tibia

Action

Inversion of the foot at subtalar joint
Plantarflexion of foot at talocrural joint
Stabilization of small movements at the ankle
Helps to control eversion of the foot at subtalar joint and dorsiflexion of foot at talocrural joint when eccentrically contracted

Nerve supply

Tibial nerve
L4, L5, S1

Arterial supply

Posterior tibial artery

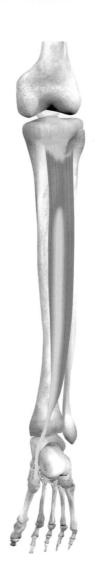

Clinical facts

Works synergistically with flexor hallucis longus, flexor digitorum longus.

Posterior tibialis is a major stabilizer of the ankle and prevents over-pronation during walking.

Tibialis posterior further supports the medial longitudinal arch of the foot.

A good learning mnemonic for the structures that pass behind the medial malleolus is: "Tom, Dick an' Harry" (Tibialis posterior, flexor Digitorum longus, posterior tibial Artery, tibial Nerve, flexor Hallucis longus).

Palpation

1. Performed prone.
2. Place palpating fingers over fibers on posterior calf.
3. Instruct the client to invert and plantarflex the ankle.
4. Note the contraction within the muscle tissue. Remember to palpate deep to the gastrocnemius/soleus from origin to insertion behind the medial malleolus to sole of foot.

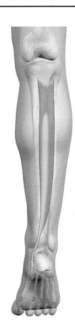

Manual muscle test

Position

Performed supine with ankle plantarflexed and inverted.

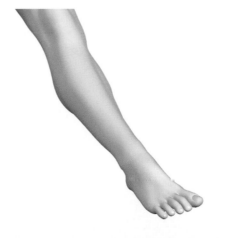

Test

Examiner applies a resistance force on the foot diagonally from the medial to lateral and toward dorsiflexion.

Use an appropriate grading scale to record the findings. Remember to test through the range.

A midrange test can be used to assess isometric strength, wherein the client is instructed to hold the position without a resistant force being applied by the examiner.

Stabilization

Examiner can stabilize the movement by placing a supporting hand laterally above the ankle.

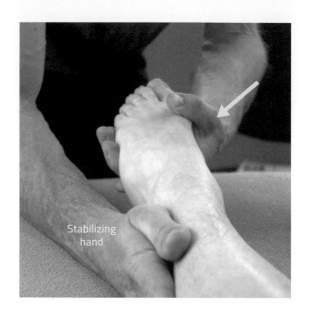

Stabilizing hand

Kinesiology muscle test

Position

Performed supine. Client's foot is fully plantarflexed and inverted. (DOWN AND IN)

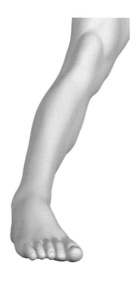

Test

Client is instructed to hold this position. Examiner grasps the foot with both hands, so any movement of the client only occurs at the ankle. Examiner moves slightly, exerting a light pressure on the foot, as if to take the foot back to the neutral position.

Stabilization

Examiner holds the foot with two hands, isolating the ankle joint as the only joint at which movement will occur.

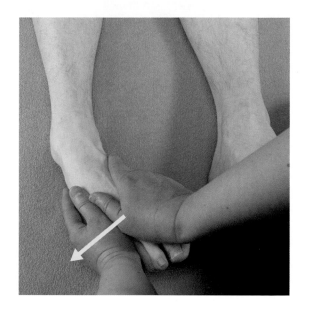

Kinesiological associations

Organ: Bladder
Acupuncture meridian: Urinary bladder
Emotion: Fear

Video: Tibialis posterior

FIBULARIS GROUP (peroneus)

This lateral group of leg muscles is often referred to as the peroneal or fibularis group, because of the attachments and close association with the fibula. The group comprises the following muscles: fibularis (peroneus) tertius, longus, and brevis.

Origin

Fibularis tertius
Distal third of anterior portion of fibula
Fibularis longus
Head and proximal lateral shaft of fibula
Fibularis brevis
Distal two thirds of lateral fibula

Insertion

Fibularis tertius
Base of 5th metatarsal
Fibularis longus
Medial cuneiform and base of 1st metatarsal
Fibularis brevis
Tuberosity of 5th metatarsal

Action

Fibularis tertius
Dorsiflexion of foot at talocrural joint
Eversion of foot at subtalar joint
Fibularis longus and brevis
Eversion of foot at subtalar joint
Plantarflexion of foot at talocrural joint
Helps to control inversion of foot at subtalar joint and dorsiflexion of foot at talocrural joint when eccentrically contracted

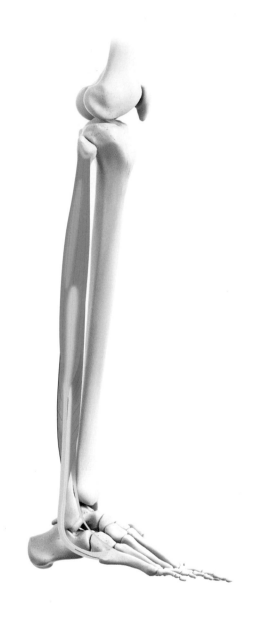

Nerve supply
Superficial peroneal nerve
L4, L5, S1

Arterial supply
Peroneal artery

Clinical facts

Fibularis (peroneus) longus and brevis work synergistically for eversion and plantarflexion of foot, and gastrocnemius and soleus for plantarflexion.
Fibularis longus and brevis pass behind the lateral malleolus with fibularis tertius passing in front, thus working predominantly as a plantarflexor.

The fibularis group together with tibialis anterior constitute the stirrup of the foot. Fibularis longus is a key stabilizer of the ankle and helps to balance the force of the ankle invertors. Fibularis longus often requires strength-related rehabilitation in patients who have chronic ankle instability and inversion sprains.

Palpation

1. Client is supine or seated.
2. Place palpating fingers over fibularis fibers anterior to the lateral malleolus.
3. Instruct the client to evert the ankle.
4. Note the contraction within the muscle tissue. Remember to palpate from insertion to origin.

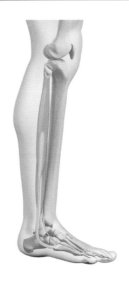

Manual muscle test

Position

Fibularis tertius
Performed supine, with ankle dorsiflexed and everted.

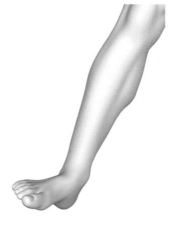

Fibularis tertius

Fibularis longus and brevis
Performed supine, with ankle plantarflexed
and everted.

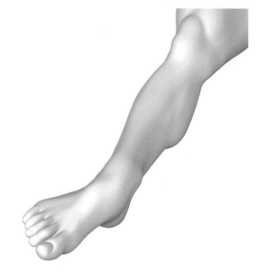

Fibularis longus and brevis

Test

Fibularis tertius
Examiner applies a resistance force
diagonally from the lateral to medial and
toward plantarflexion.

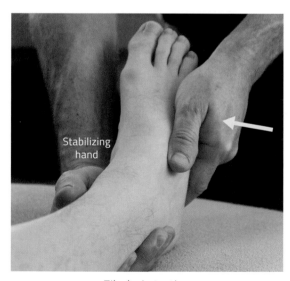

Stabilizing
hand

Fibularis tertius

Fibularis longus and brevis

Examiner applies a resistance force in a rotational pattern from lateral to medial and into dorsiflexion.

Use an appropriate grading scale to record the findings. Remember to test through the range.

A midrange test can be used to assess isometric strength, wherein the client is instructed to hold the position without a resistant force being applied by the examiner.

Stabilization

Examiner can stabilize the movement by placing a supporting hand anteriorly above the ankle.

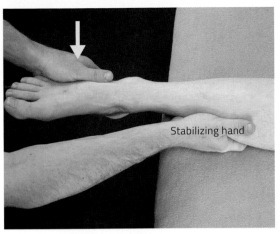

Stabilizing hand

Fibularis longus and brevis

Kinesiology muscle test

Position

Fibularis tertius
Performed supine with full dorsiflexion and
eversion of foot. (UP AND OUT)

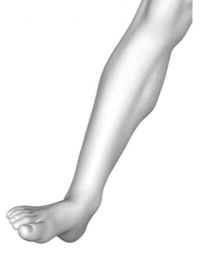

Fibularis tertius

Fibularis longus and brevis
Performed supine with full plantarflexion
and eversion of foot. (DOWN AND OUT)

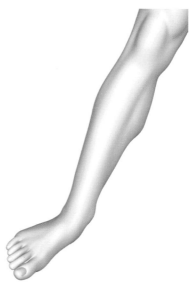

Fibularis longus and brevis

Test

Client is instructed to hold this position. Examiner grasps the foot with both hands, so any movement of the client only occurs at the ankle. Examiner moves slightly, exerting a light pressure on the foot, as if to take the foot back to the neutral position.

Stabilization

Examiner holds the foot with two hands, isolating the ankle joint as the only joint at which movement will occur.

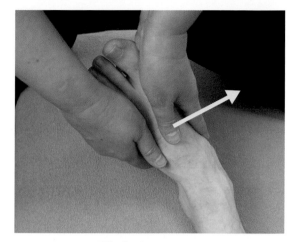

Fibularis tertius

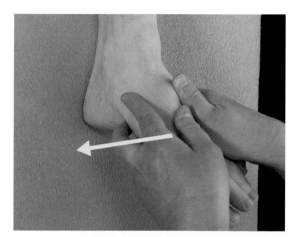

Fibularis longus and brevis

Kinesiological associations

Organ: Bladder
Acupuncture meridian: Urinary bladder
Emotion: Fear

Video: Fibularis longus and brevis

EXTENSOR HALLUCIS LONGUS

Origin

Anterior middle third of fibula and interosseous membrane

Insertion

Base of distal phalanx of the big toe

Action

Extends big toe and assists with foot dorsiflexion and inversion
Helps to control flexion of big toe if eccentrically contracted

Nerve supply

Deep peroneal nerve
L4, L5, S1

Arterial supply

Anterior tibial artery

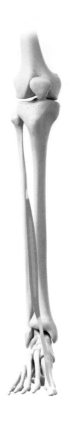

Clinical facts

Works synergistically with extensor hallucis brevis and tibialis anterior.
The muscle controls deceleration of the forefoot, after heel strike during the gait cycle.

The dorsalis pedis artery is palpable on the anterior surface of the ankle between the tendons of extensor hallucis longus and extensor digitorum longus.

Palpation

1. Client is supine or seated.
2. Place palpating fingers over the fibers lateral to the anterior distal tibia.
3. Instruct the client to extend the big toe by bringing big toe toward the anterior shin.
4. Note the contraction within the muscle tissue. Remember to palpate from insertion to origin.

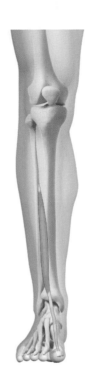

Manual muscle test

Position

Supine, with ankle in a neutral position and big toe fully extended.

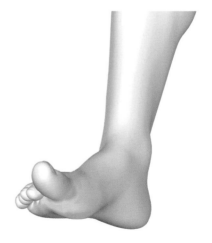

Test

Examiner applies a resistance force toward flexion of the big toe.

Use an appropriate grading scale to record the findings. Remember to test through the range.

A midrange test can be used to assess isometric strength, wherein the client is instructed to hold the position without a resistant force being applied by the examiner.

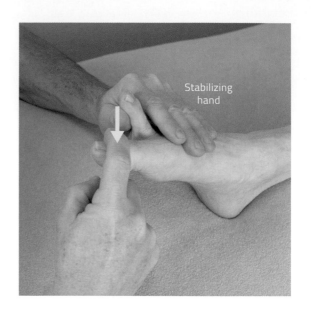

Stabilization

Place a supporting hand over the dorsal surface of 2nd to 5th phalanges.

Kinesiology muscle test

Position

Supine, with ankle in neutral position. Big toe is partially extended to 45°.

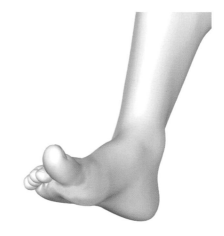

Test

Client is instructed to hold this position whilst the examiner gently rocks their body exerting a light force on the big toe, moving it toward flexion.

Stabilization

Standing beside the foot being tested, lightly support the foot with the other hand, making sure that no movement occurs in the rest of the foot and ankle.

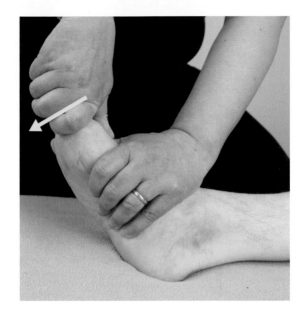

Kinesiological associations

Not known

Video: Extensor hallucis longus

FLEXOR HALLUCIS LONGUS

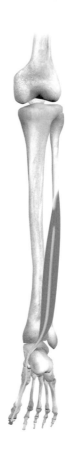

Origin

Posterior inferior two thirds of fibula and interosseous membrane

Insertion

Base of distal phalanx of plantar surface of big toe

Action

Flexion of big toe (bringing toward plantarflexion as if curling toes under)
Assists with plantarflexion and inversion of foot
Helps to control extension of big toe when eccentrically contracted

Nerve supply

Tibial nerve
L5, S1, S2

Arterial supply

Posterior tibial artery

Clinical facts

Works synergistically with flexor hallucis brevis.
The muscle is relatively large and works to produce a propulsive force during the push-off and toe-off phases of the gait cycle.

When toe abnormalities exist, such as hallux valgus (a laterally deviated big toe), the efficiency of flexor hallucis longus is reduced. Flexor hallucis longus further maintains the medial longitudinal arches of the foot.

Palpation

1. Performed prone.
2. Place palpating fingers over the fibers of the distal posterior calf.
3. Instruct the client to flex the big toe.
4. Note the contraction within the muscle tissue. Remember to palpate deep to the triceps surae from origin to insertion, posteriorly to the medial malleolus following a line to the sole of the foot.

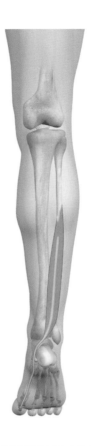

Manual muscle test

Position

Supine, with ankle in a neutral position and big toe fully flexed.

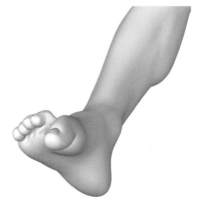

Test

Examiner applies a resistance force toward extension of the big toe.

Stabilization

Place a supporting hand over the 2nd to 5th phalanges.

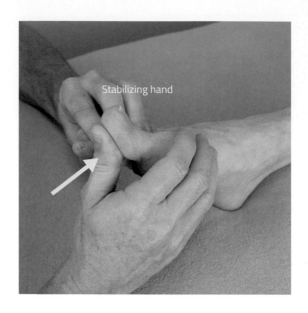

Kinesiology muscle test

Position

Supine, with ankle in a neutral position and big toe partially flexed to 45° (as if curling big toe under).

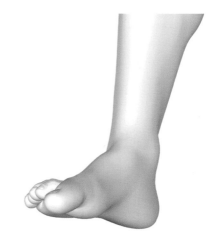

Test

Client is instructed to hold this position whilst examiner gently rocks their body, exerting a light force on the big toe, moving it toward extension (as if dorsiflexing just the big toe).

Stabilization

Standing beside the foot being tested, lightly support the foot with the other hand, making sure that no movement occurs in the rest of the foot and ankle.

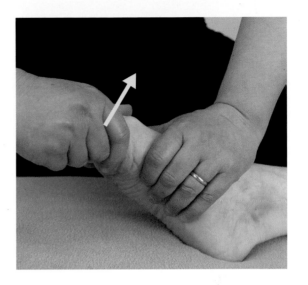

Kinesiological associations

Organ: Reproductive and endocrine organs
Acupuncture meridian: Circulation/sex
Emotion: Various, depending on which organs are affected

Video: Flexor hallucis longus

EXTENSOR DIGITORUM LONGUS

Origin

Proximal fibula, interosseous membrane, and lateral fibular condyle

Insertion

Dorsal surface of 2nd to 5th toes – via dorsal sheaths/expansions to middle and distal phalanges

Action

Extends 2nd to 5th toes at metatarsal-phalangeal and interphalangeal joints
Dorsiflexion and eversion of foot
Helps to control flexion of 2nd to 5th toes and plantarflexion and inversion of the foot when eccentrically contracted

Nerve supply

Deep peroneal nerve
L4, L5, S1

Arterial supply

Anterior tibial artery

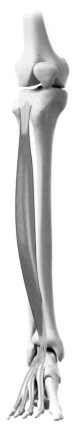

Clinical facts

Works synergistically with extensor digitorum brevis.
Extensor digitorum longus often has an additional tendon that originates from its distal muscle fibers and inserts at the base of the 5th metatarsal – this is commonly referred to as peroneus tertius.
Extensor digitorum longus assists with deceleration of the forefoot following heel strike in the gait cycle.

Palpation

1. Client is supine or seated.
2. Palpate the fibers on the dorsal surface of the foot.
3. Client is asked to extend their toes whilst resisting a force into flexion.
4. Palpate origin to insertion.
5. Look for contraction in muscle belly.

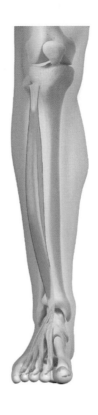

Manual muscle test

Position

Supine or seated with 2nd to 5th toes extended. Ankle should be in neutral.

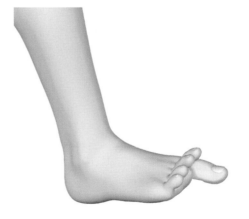

Test

A 35% resistive force is applied to encourage flexion of 2nd to 5th toes. Client is instructed to oppose the force by maintaining extension.

Stabilization

Practitioner stabilizes the big toe (hallux) to make sure it is not extended too.

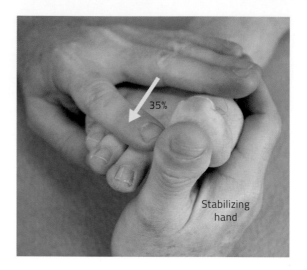

35%

Stabilizing hand

Kinesiology muscle test

Not performed

Video: Extensor digitorum longus

EXTENSOR DIGITORUM BREVIS

Origin
Proximal anterolateral aspect of calcaneus

Insertion
Distal phalanges of 2nd, 3rd, and 4th toes, via extensor digitorum longus tendons and proximal phalanx of 1st toe

Action
Extends 2nd, 3rd, and 4th toes at metatarsal-phalangeal and interphalangeal joints
Helps to control flexion of the 2nd, 3rd, and 4th toes when eccentrically contracted

Nerve supply
Deep peroneal nerve
L4, L5, S1

Arterial supply
Dorsalis pedis artery

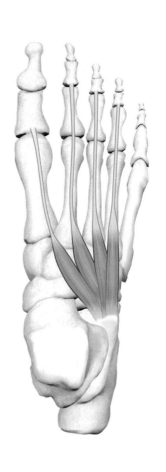

Clinical facts
Works synergistically with extensor digitorum longus.
Extensor digitorum longus and extensor hallucis brevis are the only two intrinsic muscles located on the superior aspect of the foot (dorsal surface). These two intrinsic muscles are useful clinical markers to assess edema following ankle related injury.

Palpation

1. Client is supine or seated.
2. Palpate along muscle fibers anterior to lateral malleolus.
3. Client is asked to extend their toes whilst resisting a force into flexion.
4. Palpate origin to insertion.
5. Look for contraction in muscle belly.

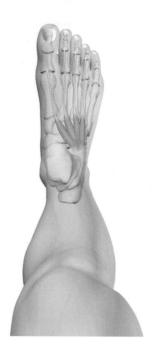

Manual muscle test

Position

Supine or seated with ankle in dorsiflexion.

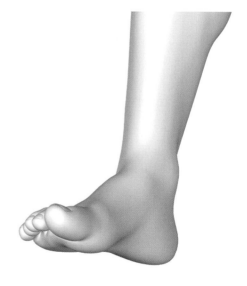

Test

A 35% resistive force is applied to encourage flexion of 2nd, 3rd, and 4th toes. Client is instructed to oppose the force by maintaining extension.

Stabilization

Practitioner stabilizes dorsal surface of foot during test.

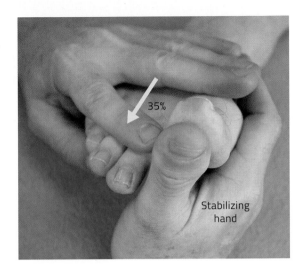

35%

Stabilizing hand

Kinesiology muscle test

Position

Supine or seated, with foot in slight plantarflexion and toes extended.

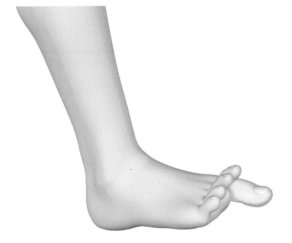

Test

Client is instructed to hold this position. Practitioner rocks their own body slightly, exerting a gentle pressure on 2nd, 3rd, and 4th toes as if to bring toes into flexion. Take care not to overpower the client.

Stabilization

Support is given at the ankle.

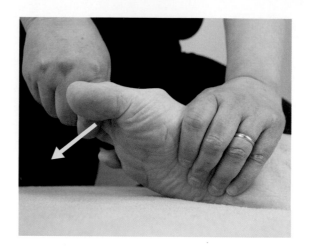

Kinesiological associations

Not known.

Video: Extensor digitorum brevis

Extensor digitorum brevis

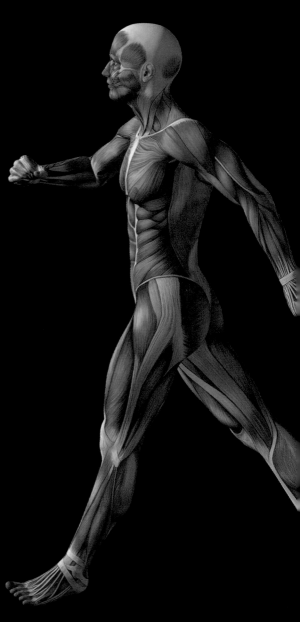

Section

3

GAIT TESTING

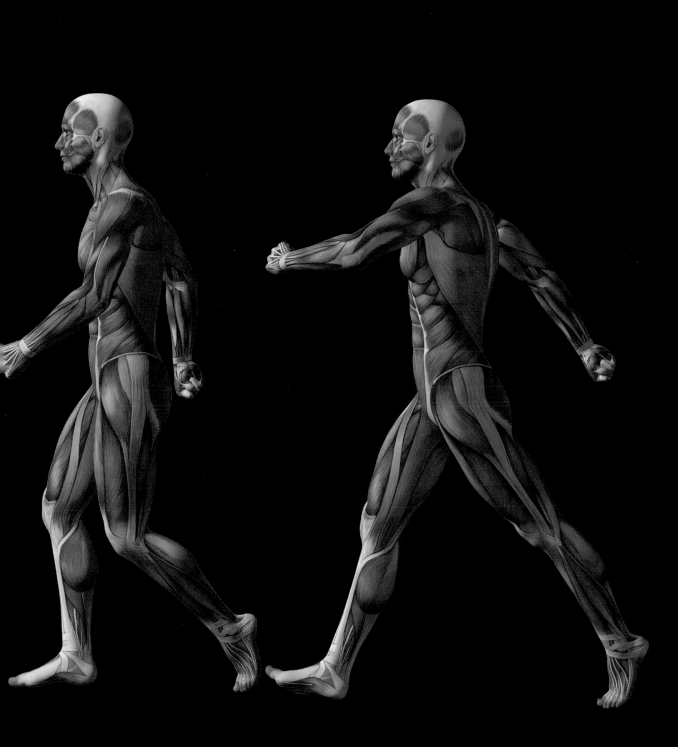

Introduction to gait testing

Gait and locomotion are complex activities using a combination of facilitation, inhibition, isometric and eccentric contraction of muscles as the body moves, balances, and breathes. All voluntary muscles are involved and are controlled by the brain, motor nerves, sensory nerves, and proprioceptors. Fascia and soft tissues change shape according to the pressures and pulls on them, and this gives a spring-like effect; the body recoils and propels itself into the shapes laid down by the ligaments and fine-tuned by muscle action.

In any controlled action, certain muscles are the major players in organizing the movement, with the other muscles being the secondary controllers of the initial movement. When crawling, walking, or running, the major muscles tend to work contralaterally. Thus, contralateral upper limbs and lower limbs are brought forward when walking. The trailing arm is contralateral to the trailing leg. For example, as the hip is flexed to bring the leg forward, the contralateral shoulder is forward flexed. Likewise, the trailing leg and contralateral arm are in hip and shoulder extension.

Several therapies, including applied kinesiology and Amatsu Soft Tissue Therapy, use combinations of muscle tests performed simultaneously to identify dysfunctional areas of the gait mechanisms. This allows clarification of the combinations of muscles which appear not to be working optimally. It does not replace observation of the client walking but offers a quick test that can be performed before and after a treatment to note any changes. Many therapists may offer prescribed activities to improve such gait function, others may treat with massage or soft tissue techniques or acupuncture/acupressure.

Although the listed tests are contralateral gait tests, all tests may be performed ipsilaterally when the client's history suggests such testing. All listed gait tests use the major muscles in the upper and lower body that initiate the walking movement being tested. They may also be used to mimic a movement that the client has expressed difficulty with, for example, walking backward or sideways. Practitioners can be creative in the use of combined muscle tests so are not limited to the listed testing methods.

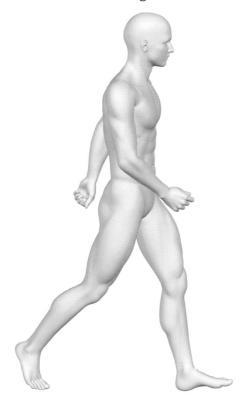

Contralateral shoulder and hip flexor gait test

This test uses the combined muscle action of all hip flexors and all shoulder flexors on the contralateral side. Both shoulder and hip flexor tests should be individually tested first to see if they are strong. If the contralateral muscles test strong individually, yet weak in combination, the gait test is thought to be a weak test.

Position

Supine, with knees and elbows fully extended. Examiner picks up the straight leg from the medial side of foot thus flexing the hip to 60° with leg abducted to shoulder width and laterally rotated. Contralateral arm is flexed to 60° with full internal rotation of humerus.

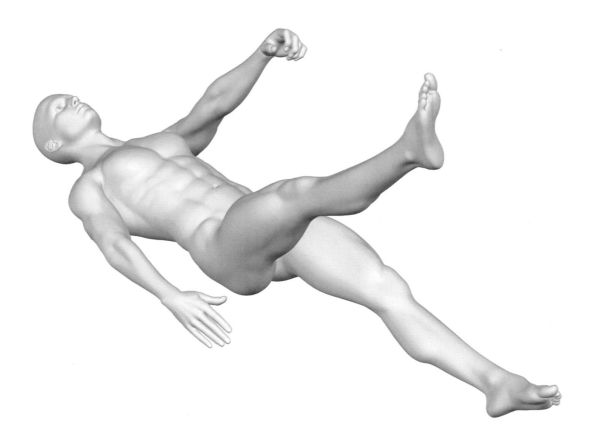

Test

Client is asked to hold that position with straight limbs. Practitioner rocks their own body slightly, exerting a light and equal pressure simultaneously on the distal portion of the lower leg and contralateral forearm. Direction of leg test is extension and slight abduction. Direction of arm test is slight abduction and toward slight shoulder extension as if to place the arm and leg back on the couch. A weak test is noted when either the leg or the arm, or both, weakens and is unable to be held in position. Most often, it is the leg that demonstrates weakness in gait testing.

Stabilization

The practitioner should stand near the treatment couch so the lower leg and forearm are both within reach. Watch for breath-holding of the client.

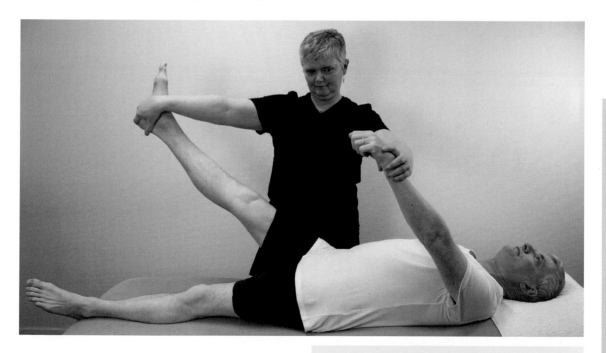

Video: Contralateral shoulder and hip flexor gait test

Contralateral shoulder and hip extensor gait test

This test uses the combined muscle action of all hip extensors and all shoulder extensors on the contralateral side. Both shoulder and hip extensor tests should be individually tested first to see if they are strong. If the contralateral muscles test strong individually, yet weak in combination, the gait test is thought to be a weak test.

Position

Prone, with knees and elbows fully extended. Hip is brought into extension and the opposite shoulder is extended to about a normal pace-length for that client.

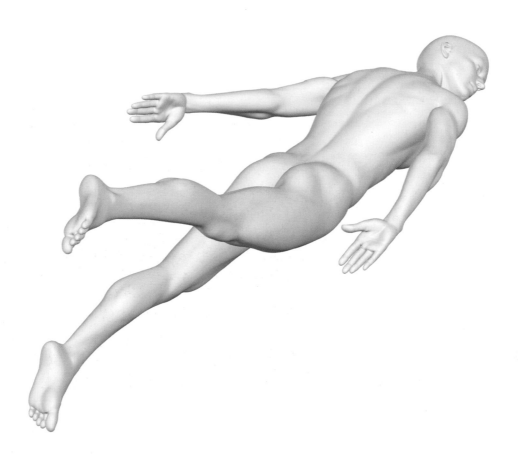

Test

Client is asked to hold that position with straight limbs. Practitioner rocks their own body slightly, exerting a light and equal pressure simultaneously on the distal portion of the lower leg and contralateral forearm, as if to return both limbs to the couch. A weak test is noted when either the leg or the arm, or both, weakens and is unable to be held in position. Most often, it is the leg that demonstrates weakness in gait testing.

Stabilization

The practitioner should stand near the treatment couch so the lower leg and forearm are both within reach. Watch for breath-holding of the client.

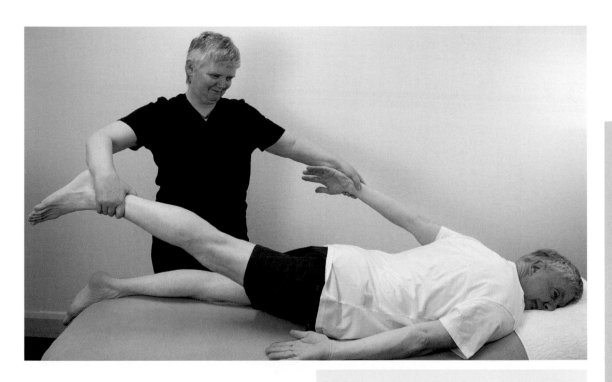

Video: Contralateral shoulder and hip extensor gait test

Contralateral shoulder and hip abductor gait test

This test uses the combined muscle action of hip abductors (mainly gluteus medius) and shoulder abductors (middle deltoid) on the contralateral side. Both shoulder and hip abductor tests should be individually tested first to see if they are strong. If the contralateral muscles test strong individually, yet weak in combination, the gait test is thought to be a weak test.

Position

Supine, with knees fully extended and elbow partially flexed. The elbow is flexed to help reach both limbs of the client. Hip is brought into abduction to approximately 30° and the opposite shoulder is abducted approximately 30°.

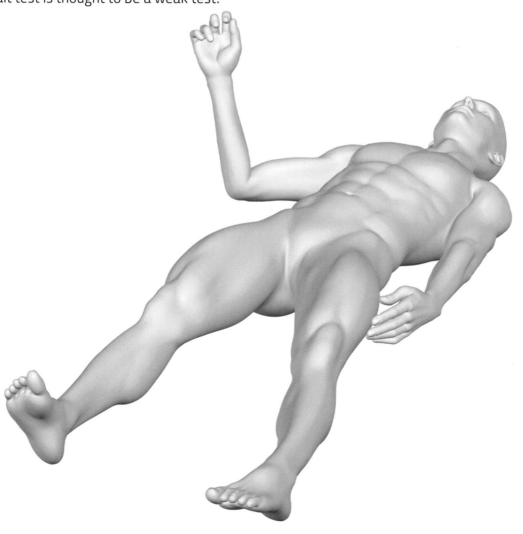

Test

Client is asked to hold that position with a straight leg. Practitioner rocks their own body slightly, exerting a light and equal pressure simultaneously on the distal portion of the lower leg and contralateral arm, as if to adduct both limbs to the body. A weak test is noted when either the leg or the arm, or both, weakens and is unable to be held in position. Most often, it is the leg that demonstrates weakness in gait testing.

Stabilization

The practitioner should stand near the treatment couch so the lower leg and forearm are both within reach. Watch for breath-holding of the client.

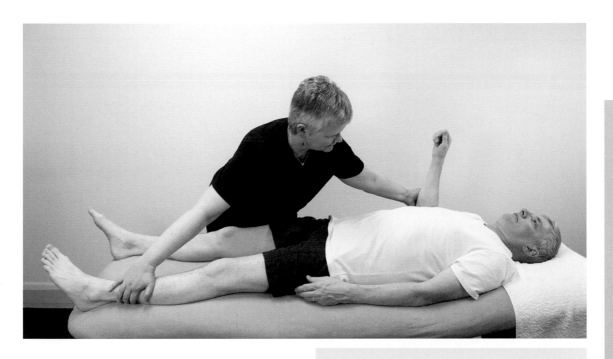

Video: Contralateral shoulder and hip abductor gait test

Contralateral shoulder and hip adductor gait test

This test uses the combined muscle action of all hip adductors and all shoulder adductors on the contralateral side. Both shoulder and hip adductor tests should be individually tested first to see if they are strong. If the contralateral muscles test strong individually, yet weak in combination, the gait test is thought to be a weak test.

Position

Supine, with knees and elbows fully extended. Hip is brought into adduction and the opposite shoulder is adducted against the body as in the latissimus dorsi test.

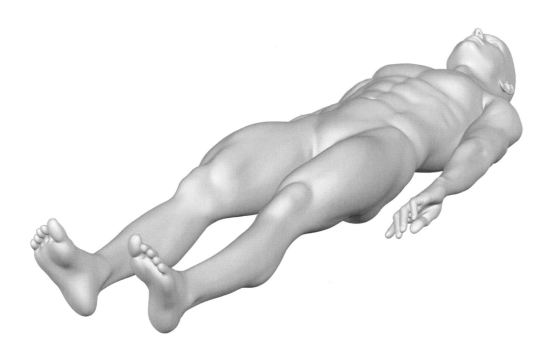

Test

Client is asked to hold that position with straight limbs. Practitioner rocks their own body slightly, exerting a light and equal pressure simultaneously on the distal portion of the lower leg and contralateral forearm, as if to abduct opposite limbs away from the midline. A weak test is noted when either the leg or the arm, or both, weakens and is unable to be held in position. Most often, it is the leg that demonstrates weakness in gait testing.

Stabilization

The practitioner should stand near the treatment couch so the lower leg and forearm are both within reach. Watch for breath-holding of the client.

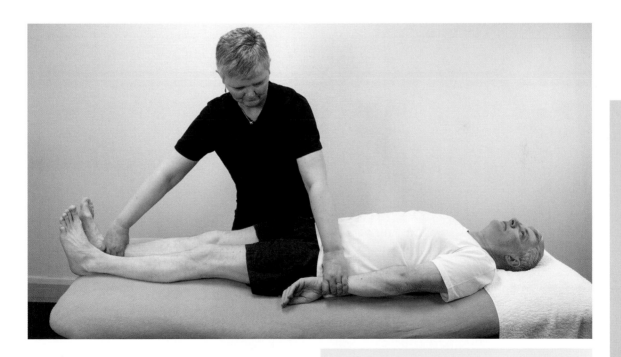

Video: Contralateral shoulder and hip adductor gait test

Contralateral shoulder and hip adductor

Contralateral psoas and pectoralis major gait test

This test uses the combined muscle action of psoas major and a modified pectoralis major test on the contralateral side. Both psoas major and pectoralis major tests should be individually tested first to see if they are strong. If the contralateral muscles test strong individually, yet weak in combination, the gait test is thought to be a weak test.

Position

Supine, with knees and elbows fully extended. Examiner picks up the straight leg from the medial side of the foot thus flexing the hip to 60° with the leg abducted to shoulder width and laterally rotated; the opposite shoulder is flexed to 60–90°, with arm fully internally rotated.

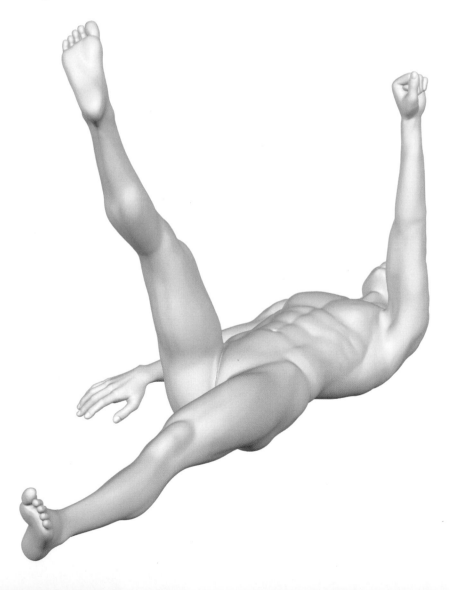

Test

Client is asked to hold that position with straight limbs. Practitioner rocks their own body slightly, exerting a light and equal pressure simultaneously on the distal portion of the lower leg and contralateral forearm, as if to return both limbs to the couch. Direction of leg test is extension and slight abduction. Direction of arm test is abduction whilst remaining in full medial rotation. A weak test is noted when either the leg or the arm, or both, weakens and is unable to be held in position. Most often, it is the leg that demonstrates weakness in gait testing.

Stabilization

The practitioner should stand near the treatment couch so the lower leg and forearm are both within reach. Watch for breath-holding of the client.

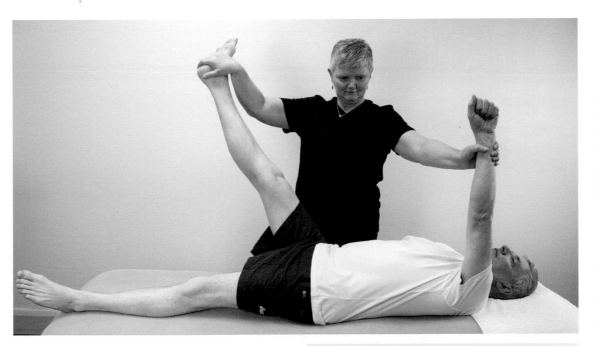

Video: Contralateral psoas and pectoralis major gait test

Contralateral gluteus medius and abdominals gait test

This test uses the combined muscle action of gluteus medius and abdominal muscles on the contralateral side. Both gluteus medius and abdominals tests should be individually tested first to see if they are strong. If the contralateral muscles test strong individually, yet weak in combination, the gait test is thought to be a weak test. Gluteus medius and abdominal muscles work to maintain support of the pelvis during walking and standing.

Position

Supine. Client crosses their forearms on their chest. Examiner picks up the straight leg and abducts to approximately shoulder width. The knee may be flexed so both limbs can be reached. Client is asked to begin to perform a sit-up or curl so the head and contralateral shoulder lift from the treatment couch, thus engaging contralateral abdominal muscles in the trunk.

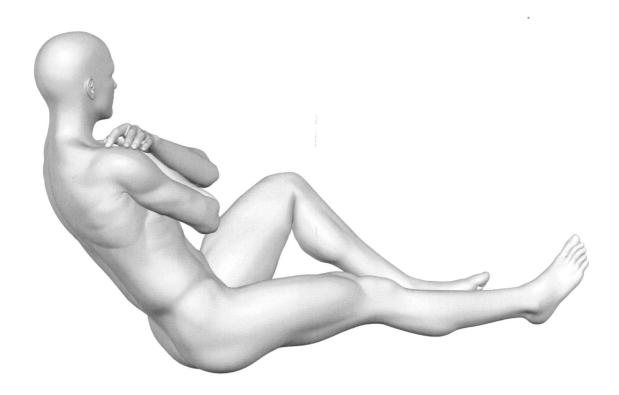

Test

Client is asked to hold that position. Practitioner rocks their own body slightly, exerting a light and equal pressure simultaneously on the distal portion of the femur in direction of adduction. A weak test is noted when either the leg weakens or the client's trunk is unable to be held in position. Timing of the test is critical; abdominal engagement must be at the same time as the gluteus medius test.

Stabilization

The practitioner should stand near the treatment couch so the lower leg and forearm are both within reach. Watch for breath-holding of the client.

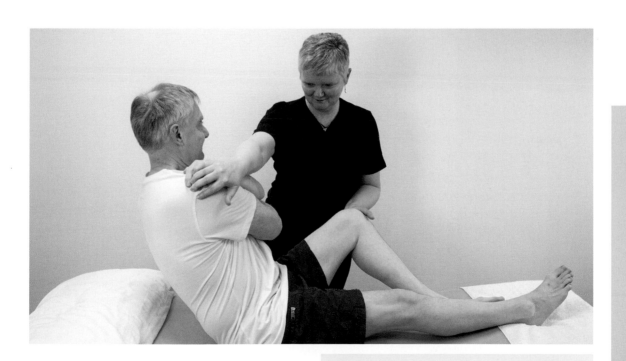

Video: Contralateral gluteus medius and abdominals gait test

Note: Page numbers followed by f indicates figures and t indicates for table respectively.